INTERMITTENT FASTING SYSTEM GUIDE

EVERYTHING YOU NEED TO KNOW ABOUT INTERMITTENT FASTING

Alice Liberti

PREFACE

Although intermittent fasting has been in many forms for thousands of years, it has only recently begun to get the answer it deserves for health and fat-loss. But what are the real health benefits of incorporating intermittent fasting into your diet and what are the side effects of fasting?

Despite of its long history, scientific studies on fasting are actually fairly rare. However, there is much empirical evidence to which some things refer. Some of those will not support you, while others are a little more unexpected. It can carry huge benefits if it is done right: weight loss, increased energy, improves blood pressure, helps the body dispose of fats and many other things. Furthermore, it can strengthen neural connections and improve memory and mood.

In this book, you will learn everything you need to know about intermittent fasting. What is clear is that in a modern society with toxins present all around, anything that can reduce their impacts must be good news for our health. After reading this book you will see that an intermittent fasting system can be easy to set up and offers real health benefits.

TABLE OF CONTENTS

CHAPTER 1

INTERMITTENT FASTING

WHAT IS INTERMITTENT FASTING ?

Fasting is a time tested and ancient tradition. It has been used not only for weight loss, but to improve concentration, extend life, prevent Alzheimers, prevent insulin resistance and even reverse the entire aging process. There is much to talk about here so we begin a new subsection "Fasting".

There is nothing new, except what has been forgotten – Marie Antoinette

So the forgotten □uestion of weight loss is "When should we eat?" We don't ignore the □uestion of frequency anywhere else. Falling from a building 1000 feet off the ground once will likely kill us. But is this the same as falling from a 1-foot wall 1000 times? Absolutely not. Yet the total distance fallen is still 1000 feet.

All foods will increase insulin levels to some degree. Eating the proper foods will prevent high levels, but won't do much to lower levels. Some foods that are better than others, but all foods still increase insulin. The key to prevention of resistance is to periodically sustain very low levels of insulin. If all foods raise insulin, then the only answer is the complete voluntary abstinence of food. The answer we are looking for is, in a word, fasting.

The answer to this vexing problem lies not in the latest and greatest diet trend, but in the tried and true. Instead of searching for some exotic, never-before-tried diet miracle, we should focus on ancient healing traditions of the past. I mean the way past. Fasting is one of the most ancient healing traditions in human history. This solution has been practiced by virtually every culture and religion on earth.

What is intermittent fasting?

Whenever fasting is mentioned, there is always the same eye-rolling response. Starvation? That's the answer? No. Fasting is completely different beast. Starvation is the involuntary absence of food. It is neither deliberate, nor controlled. Starving people have no idea when and where their next meal will come from. Fasting, on the other hand is the voluntary withholding of food for spiritual, health, or other reasons. It is the difference between suicide and dying of old age. The two terms should never be confused with each other(I will discuss about it in details below). Fasting may be done for any period of time, from a few hours to months on end. In a sense, fasting is part of everyday life. The term 'break fast' is the meal that breaks the fast – which is done daily.

Basically, intermittent fasting is a pattern of eating that alternates between periods of fasting, usually consuming only water, and non-fasting, usually eating anything a person want no matter how fattening. In other words, for example, a person can eat anything he wants during a 24-hour period and fast for the next 24 hours. This approach to weight control seems to be supported by science, as well as religious and cultural practices around the globe. Adherents of intermittent fasting claim that this practice is a way to become more circumspect about food.

If you have tried to lose weight, you probably have tried diets such as Atkins diet based on the frequent feeding theory. Simply, proponents of such diets told you to eat often during the day. The idea was that the more you eat, the faster your metabolism. The faster your metabolism, the more fat you will lose. Of course, you do know that the more you ate, the more you wanted to eat and the more your weight remained. When you are on an intermittent program, you will have to cut down your meal fre□uency. Sometimes, you have to do without breakfast.

You probably sleep for around 6 to 8 hours. During this time, your body is in fasting mode. When your body is in fasting mode, it usually produces more insulin. More insulin in your body causes your body to have increased insulin sensitivity. When your body has increased insulin sensitivity, you lose more fat. The brilliance of intermittent fasting weight loss program is that you skip breakfast to extend the period of your body's insulin sensitivity. This means that your body is going to be on fat loss mode for a longer period. You will lose more weight.

A longer fasting mode also has a good effect on the Growth hormone levels in your body. By skipping breakfast or eating during a specific period, your body produces Growth hormone. Growth hormone is what you want your body producing when you are trying to lose weight. This is simply because Growth hormone promotes weight loss in your body. When you are on an intermittent fasting weight loss program, your Growth hormone levels are usually at their peak. You will be losing more weight during this period. High Growth hormone levels in your body also have several other health benefits. This program is simply amazing!

It is important to clarify that intermittent fasting is not a diet. You are probably tired of trying anything with the word 'diet' on it when it comes to weight loss. Intermittent fasting is a way of eating that involves a structured program on the times when you eat and when you do not eat. You structure your program according to your fancy

One thing that put people off is the fear that they will be extremely hungry and not stick to the plan or do not know how to fit it into their schedule. This is actually quite simple if you plan in advance you get eat your evening meal at pretty much the same time every day but at an hour either side depending if on an intermittent fasting phase or an eating phase. Again with a little planning you can also accommodate socializing and eating out. Although this does take a little willpower and a slight degree of discomfort to begin with it is actually quite easy!

At its very core, fasting simply allows the body to burn off excess body fat. It is important to realize that this is normal and humans have evolved to fast without detrimental health consequences. Body fat is merely food energy that has been stored away. If you don't eat, your body will simply "eat" its own fat for energy.

Life is about balance. The good and the bad. The yin and the yang. The same applies to eating and fasting. Fasting, after all, is simply the flip side of eating. If you are not eating, you are fasting. When we eat, more food energy is ingested than can immediately be used. Some of this energy must be stored away for later use. Insulin is the key hormone involved in the storage of food energy. Insulin rises when we eat, helping to store the excess energy in two separate ways. Sugars can be linked into long chains, called glycogen and then stored in the liver. There is, however, limited storage space; and once that is reached, the liver starts to turn the excess glucose into fat. This process is called De-Novo Lipogenesis (meaning literally Making Fat from New).

Some of this newly created fat is stored in the liver, but most of it is exported to other fat deposits in the body. While this is a more complicated process, there is no limit to the amount of fat that can be created. So, two complementary food energy storage systems exist in our bodies. One is easily accessible but with limited storage space (glycogen), and the other is more difficult to access but has unlimited storage space (body fat).

The process goes in reverse when we do not eat (intermittent fasting). Insulin levels fall, signaling the body to start burning stored energy as no more is coming through food. Blood glucose falls, so the body must now pull glucose out of storage to burn for energy.

Glycogen is the most easily accessible energy source. It is broken down into glucose molecules to provide energy for the other cells. This can provide enough energy to power the body for 24-36 hours. After that, the body will start breaking down fat for energy.

So, that the body only really exists in two states – the fed (insulin high) state and the fasted (insulin low) state. Either we are storing food energy, or we are burning it. It's one or the other. If eating and fasting are balanced, then there is no net weight gain.

If we start eating the minute we roll out of bed, and do not stop until we go to sleep, we spend almost all our time in the fed state. Over time, we will gain weight. We have not allowed our body any time to burn food energy.

To restore balance or to lose weight, we simply need to increase the amount of time we burn food energy. That's intermittent fasting. In essence, fasting allows the body to use its stored energy. After all, that's what it is there for. The important thing to understand is that there is nothing wrong with that. That is how our bodies are designed. That's what dogs, cat, lions and bears do. That's what humans do.

A BRIEF HISTORY OF INTERMITTENT FASTING

Fasting is one of the most ancient and widespread healing traditions in the world. Hippocrates of Cos (c 460 – c370 BC) is widely considered the father of modern medicine. Among the treatments that he prescribed and championed was the practice of fasting, and the consumption of apple cider vinegar. Hippocrates wrote, "To eat when you are sick, is to feed your illness". The ancient Greek writer and historian Plutarch (cAD46 – c AD 120) also echoed these sentiments. He wrote, "Instead of using medicine, better fast today". Ancient Greek thinkers Plato and his student Aristotle were also staunch supporters of fasting. Fasting was also ritualised in many aspects of Christianity and Judaism, and became the fourth of the five pillars of Islam. Religious fasting was intertwined with ritual and spiritual discipline, and became a form of penitence and identification with the poor and unfortunate.

The ancient Greeks believed that medical treatment could be observed from nature. Humans, like most animals, do not eat when they become sick. For this reason, fasting has been called the 'physician within'. This fasting 'instinct' that makes dogs, cats and humans anorexic when sick. This sensation is certainly familiar to everybody. Consider the last time you were sick with the flu. Probably the last thing you wanted to do was eat. So, fasting seems to be a universal human instinct to multiple forms of illnesses. Thus fasting is ingrained into human heritage, and as old as mankind itself.

The ancient Greeks believed that fasting improves cognitive abilities. Think about the last time you ate a huge Thanksgiving meal. Did you feel more energetic and mentally alert afterwards? Or, instead did you feel sleepy and a little dopey? More likely the latter. Blood is shunted to your digestive system to cope with the huge influx of food, leaving less blood going to the brain. Result – food coma.

Other intellectual giants were also great proponents of fasting. Philip Paracelsus, the founder of toxicology and one of three fathers of modern Western medicine (along with Hippocrates and

Galen) wrote, "Fasting is the greatest remedy – the physician within". Benjamin Franklin (1706-1790), one of the America's founding fathers and renowned for wide knowledge in many areas once wrote of fasting "The best of all medicines is resting and fasting".

When history meets modern research

An interesting angle of looking at the problem of intermittent feeding/fasting was employed by Panda and his colleagues, of the Salk Institute. Most of our bodily functions throughout the day are controlled by a master pacemaker situated in a brain structure called the SCN (for supra chiasmatic nucleus). This pacemaker gets neural signals from the eyes and is, thus, controlled primarily by the light/dark periods. But in a similar arrangement to our Federal system, every organ has its own sub-pacemaker, designed to serve the specific re□uirements of that organ.

In the liver, Panda et al. found that when they withheld food from mice for 24 hours, 90% of the genes that are under the circadian regulation of the clock ceased to function. Not surprisingly, since one would expect the major metabolic organ to be controlled by the supply of food. On the other hand, let mice eat a high-fat diet 24 hours a day and all the

genes under the control of the liver circadian
pacemaker get activated around the clock.
Unsurprisingly, the mice became obese.

How does this translate into humans?

One approach has been to examine pockets of
exceptional longevity in the world, a well-known one
being the Okinawa Island of Japan. These elders are
known to practice the Japanese dictum of hara hachi
bu (eat until 80% full), but it is not known whether
this is the reason that there are more centenarians here
per 100,000 residents than elsewhere in the world.
The maximum life span has not however been
extended in Okinawans. Studies of intermittent
fasting in humans, such as the CALERIE study, have
been relatively short–term and have shown benefits
on health in terms of lower weight, cardiovascular
risk factors, and diabetes risk, but the studies have so
far mostly recruited overweight people. In another
fascinating experiment, eight volunteers lived for two
years in a Biosphere – a 3 acre enclosed ecological
mini-world – and inadvertently suffered CR. Their
weight reduced by about 20%, and there were marked
reductions in blood pressure, fasting blood glucose,

insulin, cholesterol, thyroid hormone and white blood
cells. The message – we cannot be sure that the
overall lifespan will increase but IF is likely to
produce significant health benefits and increase the
likelihood of reaching the maximum potential age in a
relatively healthy state, including a healthy brain
without dementia.

Intermittent fasting is not starvation

The big misconception about fasting and starvation
is that they're the same thing. Although they might
seem very similar, they're actually distinctive
metabolic states. There's quite a significant difference
between them. They're almost like day and night.

Fasting is the complete abstention from food in
any shape or form. Usually, people still drink water
and other non-caloric beverages. It's voluntary and
controlled. You've planned it and are doing it because
you've decided to do so.

Starvation, on the other hand, is described as the
absence of essential nutrients that could support the
life of an organism. Whenever the body can't get
access to fuel or has run out of it, then it begins to
slowly die and waste away. This is irrational and

involuntary. It's forced upon and not something you choose.

The difference between fasting and starvation is like the difference between suicide and dying of old age. One is deliberate and carefully orchestrated, whereas the other is something that simply happens to you without you being able to do anything about it. Of course, here fasting resembles suicide because it's self-imposed, but it's not going to end with death. The idea remains.

You're Either One or the Other

Abstention from food is the art of manipulating our metabolic system and can be done for many reasons. Malpractice might look like the person is starving, but if done correctly it's very healthy and good for you.

Our body can only be in 2 metabolic states

Fasted – meaning that there are no exogenous calories consumed at all.
Fed – there is some food circulating the bloodstream.

Even consuming small amounts of food will put you into a fed state. It doesn't matter whether you eat

200 calories or 1000, you'll still inhibit autophagy and be shifted out of a fasted state.

That's why intermittent fasting is a lot better than caloric restriction. If you're feeding yourself, but in inadequate amounts, then your body will most definitely perceive it as scarcity. You'll be causing more damage than good. If you do it the wrong way, you'll end up like someone from the concentration camps.

How does Fasting Changes the Metabolism

Long periods of daily caloric restriction decrease the metabolism, so it's easy to presume that this would be magnified as food intake drops to zero. However, this is wrong. Once your food intake stops completely (you start to fast), the body shifts into using stored fat for fuel (ketosis). The hormonal adaptations of fasting will not occur by only lowering your caloric intake. In the case of being fasted, your physiology is under completely different conditions, which is unachievable by regular eating.

Starvation happens when there is not enough nutrition to be found e.g. when you go on a weight loss diet and restrict calories. While fasting, the organism is almost never deprived of essential nutrients, unless you lose all of your body fat. These fuel sources are mobilized from internal resources.

Fasting isn't a mechanism of starvation because your metabolism will be altered. This shift won't occur entirely if you continue consuming food, even when you've reduced your calories to a bare minimum. It's actually a lot healthier way of losing weight, as you'll be burning only fat, not muscle. When on a restrictive diet you'll never make the leap and to keep your energy demands at a balance you begin to cannibalize your own tissue. When in a fasted state, this can be circumvented.

The hormonal reactions that occur while fasting can actually make the body more nourished than while eating. In response to the disappearance of calories, we will trigger some of the most powerful anabolic hormones within us, that lead to some serious adaptations that reduce the loss of muscle almost entirely.

Fasting Doesn't Deprive You Of Nutrients

There's no reason to be concerned about malnutrition during fasting either because our fat stores can deposit almost an infinite amount of calories. The main issue is rather micronutrient deficiencies. Potassium levels may drop slightly, but even 2 months of fasting don't decrease it below a safe margin. Magnesium, calcium, and phosphorus remain stable because 99% of them are stored in our bones.

The longest recorded fast lasted for 382 days (1 year and almost 1 month). It was done by a 27-year old obese man, who lost 125 kg (276 lb) in the process. After that much time, did he even know how food tasted like? Imagine that first bite…The researchers managed to sustain such a long period with no harmful effects on the man's health thanks to taking a simple multivitamin. Of course, he was severely overweight and had a ton of extra body fat to burn, but you can be very well nourished for a long time by having access to enough micronutrients.

Intermittent Fasting and Feasting

As mentioned earlier, our metabolism can only be in either a fed or a fasted state. One involves the complete abstention from food, whereas the other can be triggered by any amounts. The degree of how fed we are dictates whether we're in starvation mode or not.

Fasting would only become dangerous when the body has completely run out of its endogenous nutrients, which would take a long time. Eventually, it can turn into starvation. Doing it intermittently, just enough, is actually extremely healthy and empowering.

I practice some form of intermittent fasting every single day. Restricting my feeding window enables me to trigger some of the most powerful anabolic hormones and metabolic process within our body. Coupling that with feasting leads to some serious adaptations that help me to build muscle, burn fat, live longer and be happier.

Intermittent Fasting — More a Lifestyle Than a Diet

I have been experimenting with different types of scheduled eating for the past two years and currently restrict my eating to a 6- to 7-hour window each day. While you're not required to restrict the amount of food you eat when on this type of daily scheduled eating plan, I would caution against versions of intermittent fasting that gives you free reign to eat all the junk food you want when not fasting, as this seems awfully counterproductive.

Also, according to research published in 2010, 2 intermittent fasting with compensatory overeating did not improve survival rates nor delay prostate tumor growth in mice. Essentially, by gorging on non-fasting days, the health benefits of fasting can easily be lost. If so, then what's the point? I view intermittent fasting as a lifestyle, not a diet, and that includes making healthy food choices whenever you do eat. Also, proper nutrition becomes even more important when fasting, so you really want to address your food choices before you try fasting.

This includes minimizing carbs and replacing them with healthful fats, like coconut oil, olive oil, olives, butter, eggs, avocados, and nuts. It typically takes several weeks to shift to fat burning mode, but once you do, your cravings for unhealthy foods and carbs will automatically disappear. This is because you're now actually able to burn your stored fat and don't have to rely on new fast-burning carbs for fuel. Unfortunately, despite mounting evidence, many health practitioners are still reluctant to prescribe fasting to their patients. According to Brad Pilon, author of Eat Stop Eat;

"Health care practitioners across the board are so afraid to recommend eating less because of the stigma involved in that recommendation, but we are more than happy to recommend that someone start going to the gym. If all I said was you need to get to the gym and start eating healthier, no one would have a problem with it. When the message is not only should you eat less, but you could probably go without eating for 24 hours once or twice a week, suddenly it's heresy."

However, the real point is that intermittent fasting does not involve starving for days on end, but rather works in harmony with the body's normal circadian rhythms. It is more of a lifestyle rather than diet.

CHAPTER 2

METHODS OF INTERMITTENT FASTING

Intermittent fasting is different for everyone. The general concept of intermittent fasting works like this: you eat almost whatever you want for a certain period of time, and then for a given amount of time you try not to consume anything other than water, tea, black coffee, and other non-caloric liquids.

It sounds pretty simple, but there are actually a few different types of intermittent fasting to choose from. Of course, everyone is different. So it's important you choose a plan that best fits your needs, your lifestyle, and your goals. It does come with a small caveat, however, and it is that you have to be in a caloric deficit in order to begin losing weight and inches off your waistline. While some have difficulty fasting through extended periods, others walk through it like a breeze. Luckily, intermittent fasting is a concept that allows you to go your own pace.

You may want to ease yourself into it over a long period of time until you are so used to intermittent fasting that it becomes second nature, or you could dare to jump right into its toughest iterations and see if you have the mental strength to overcome intense hunger pangs.

If you are looking to get into intermittent fasting and need a good place to start, I have detailed some of the eating and fasting schedules people have come up with all over the world. In this chapter, I will share the six different types of intermittent fasting schedules you can try today and you can find the one that best fits your lifestyle.

Fasting Within a Daily Window (8:16)

This is often the most popular way of intermittent fasting since it's easier for us to naturally eat this way. For example, someone might skip breakfast and have their first meal at noon, then eat regularly throughout the rest of the day but stop eating at 8pm. This means you'd be eating for an 8-hour period and fasting for 16 hours.

These times are just an example, too. Some people might prefer to start eating later in the day (works especially well for those who are used to skipping breakfast), while others will start earlier and have an early dinner.

The amount of time for this varies. Some people will eat within a small timeframe, such as six-, four-, or even one-hour period, eating only one big meal per day. What's important to remember here is that no matter when you do eat during the day, you should still get your day's worth of calories and be mindful of macro and micronutrient needs. Most people see the greatest success, and do so healthfully, with this method when sticking to a regular feeding time schedule and making it fit with your lifestyle.

The 16:8 intermittent fasting

It is the first stage in a long journey ahead. It poses a challenge for those who have never fasted before or those who particularly like eating breakfast or dinner. This is the point where you have to give up one of those two meals. Fasting for 16 hours, which includes your 8 hours of sleep, and then feeding for 8 hours, takes some time to get used to. It usually takes around 2-3 weeks to get a good grasp of for beginners and those who have never fasted.

If you have your last meal by 8 o'clock in the evening and then sleep at 10 every night and wake up at 6, that's 10 solid hours of fasting already. Skipping breakfast, 16:8 will then have you take in your first meal at exactly 12 noon. It can be tough at first, but it gets easier after a while. Make sure to keep yourself well-hydrated during your fasting window.

The '5:2' fast allots five days for eating and two days for restriction.

The 5:2 intermittent fasting diet works by allotting you five days a week to eat whatever you want, and restricting your diet for two days to 500 calories or less. These two days of fasting don't have to be one right after the other but are instead intermixed throughout the week to give your body time to recover. But on the non-fasting days, you're encouraged to eat how you normally eat. Many findings has reported that the 5:2 diet may have several impressive health benefits, including weight loss, reduced insulin resistance and decreased inflammation.

Alternate Days Fasting

This method involves fasting for a few days each week and eating as you normally would for the other days. For example, you could fast on Monday and Wednesday and eat normally the rest of the days out of your week. Another version of this is the 5-2 method discussed above: eating normally five days out of the week and choosing two days to eat around ¼ of your regular caloric intake (which is usually

around 500-600 calories for the average person), only
that alternate-day fasting its more of a routine, daily
occurrence.

Fasting on alternate days can be really flexible for
most people and lets you customize your week. In a
small study with 24 women, the 5-2 method was even
found to help protect against breast cancer. It is good
to note that simply restricting calories for days might
be harder than just fasting for some people, plus
there's no guarantee it will put you into ketosis. The
□uality of the food definitely matters, so unless you
focus on whole, low-carb foods, the low calorie days
can be really uncomfortable. Research has reported
that alternate-day fasting may "reduce waist
circumference, decrease blood pressure, lower LDL
cholesterol and decrease blood triglycerides."

The warrior diet

It is another extreme form of intermittent fasting
but comes with a bit more flexibility in the eyes of
some participants. With this form, you fast for about
20 hours a day, eating only raw fruits and vegetables
as well as drinking non-caloric li□uids. And then at
the end of the day, within a four-hour window, you
eat a big meal. If you're focusing on keto foods,
obviously you'd want to forgo the fruit and focus on
low-carb vegetables and keto snacks.

Since small snacks are "allowed" before evening, it can be easier than forgoing food altogether during the day. Some people might also like eating a lot at night. Plus, this system promotes high-□uality foods choices and staying away from added sugars and processed foods.

Erratic "anything goes" hunger-centered fasting.

This becomes a broad category open to massive interpretation, unless you really learn to listen to your body. Basically, you eat when you're hungry and abstain when you're not. You don't just eat because it's lunchtime, for example. Proponents of this type of fasting suggest eating sensibly most of the time, eating nothing for an extended period every now and then, and indulging occasionally. This "anything goes" IF perspective works best when a health care professional custom-designs a plan for you rather than you whimsically deciding when to eat or not. Its flexibility, however, becomes ideal during vacations and other occasions when you know you'll eat less-than-healthy foods.

When it comes to IF, there is no one plan that work for everyone. Figuring out what works for you takes some trial-and-error, and a professional can help you tweak and troubleshoot. If you do it alone, I suggest starting with a simple form that best suits your lifestyle. As we have discovered, immediately leaping into a more challenging plan could have unpleasant side effects. Remember, there are also a few caveat. Fasting for longer periods of time when your body isn't prepared can yield serious consequences. If you feel lightheaded or weak, eat something. Fasting isn't a magical "cure-all"; it's simply another tool in your weight-loss and optimal-health arsenal.

No matter what method you use, the "rules" are pretty similar: During fasting times, plan to only drink water, black coffee, or other beverages without added sugars or calories, such as unsweetened iced or herbal teas. This will not only help you stay hydrated but also help reduce feelings of hunger. Even though fasting is great and healthy, it's really important to eat high-quality foods during your feeding times, especially if weight loss and/or ketosis is your goal. I will discuss this in the coming chapter and you will see my list of ketogenic foods to help you stay in ketosis, and always remember to regularly test your ketone levels.

Intermittent Fasting With Diet Fads - Why It Works Better

People experiencing intermittent fasting have proved that it does not cause starvation, tiredness, and other symptoms of daily diet. It is because it is not the same with diet fad. It is completely different with completely different results.

Everyone already knows diet as a general way of losing fat. It is free of charge, simple and easy. However, the result it gives is not even if compared to the hard work someone must go through in dieting. Surely diet will help in losing weight but it will not be a drastic change, and this change will probably take place after a few weeks of dieting. This is where the difference lies between diet and intermittent fasting. Following a flexible short-term fasting will give an incredible result.

Not only will it reduce weight fast but also show a drastic change in the body. This method affects the lifestyle of those doing the weight loss program. So, it can be a long lasting weight loss program. Another difference is the phrase 'burn fat feed muscle' applies in intermittent fasting. Many people have proved while following this type of method they did not lose any muscle mass.

Knowing the differences leads to a conclusion. Based on the facts given, intermittent fasting is one step ahead in succeeding to weight loss compared to diet fad. Succeeding in the results and also the process. It is a lifetime program which is far from regrettable.

Should You Do Intermittent Fasting and the Keto Diet?

By only eating fat and protein, your body must adapt to run on fat for fuel instead of carbohydrates. In the absence of carbs/glucose, your body converts fats to ketones and uses them for fuel. This process is called "ketosis," and there are two ways for a body to enter ketosis:

Eating in a way that induces ketosis (very low carb, high fat).

Fasting…Hey, that's what you're reading about right now!

As many will tell you: Eating Keto + Intermittent Fasting = a great combo for simple weight loss.

Here's how the fasting portion of it works:

As your body enters a fast period when there are no sources of glucose energy readily available, the liver begins the process of breaking down fat into ketones. Fasting itself can trigger ketosis. Fasting for a period of time before kicking off a Keto-friendly eating plan could speed your transition into the metabolic state of ketosis, and fasting intermittently while in ketosis could help you maintain that state.

I personally love fasting for the simplicity: I skip breakfast every day and train in a fasted state. It's one less decision I have to make, it's one less opportunity to make a bad food choice, and it helps me reach my goals.

WHY KETO + IF WORKS = eating Keto can be really challenging. And every time you eat, it's an opportunity to do it wrong and accidentally eat foods that knock you out of ketosis. You're also tempted to overeat. So, by skipping a meal, you're eliminating one meal, one decision, one chance to screw up.

Your value may vary!

You need to decide what works for you. You probably won't become "keto-adapted" (your body running on ketones) just skipping breakfast every day – your body will still have enough glucose stored from your carb-focused meals for lunch and dinner the day before.

In order to use fasting to enter ketosis, the fast needs to be long enough to deplete your carb/glucose stores, or you need to severely restrict carbohydrates from your meals in addition to IF in order to enter ketosis.

Experiment and try different strategies that will work for you. By skipping a meal or minimizing carbohydrate intake, you're more likely than not to lose weight.

You can do intermittent fasting without eating a Keto Diet and lose weight. You can do a Keto Diet without intermittent Fasting and lose weight. You can combine them and lose weight. Any of those options could work for you, but you need to make it work for your lifestyle!

CHAPTER 3

WHAT TO EAT AND DRINK DURING INTERMITTENT FASTING

Limiting your daily calorie intake is associated with an extended intermittent fasting span. So, the buzzy concept behind intermittent fasting is actually nothing we haven't already heard before. Intermittent fasting, or IF, is not actually considered a diet, but rather a eating pattern. And as discussed earlier, it has been proven to promote healthy brain function, lower blood sugar, and help maintain a healthy body weight. And the best part is you supposedly can eat what you want during your allotted amount of time during the day. it's no wonder that everyone you know seems to be jumping on the IF bandwagon. Maybe the appeal is the lack of food rules. There are restrictions on when you can eat, but not necessarily what you can eat. So should you be downing pints of ice cream and bags of chips while intermittent fasting? Probably not. That's why I 've come up with a list of the best foods to include in your IF life.

Eating the wrong foods during your meal times can counter the benefits of intermittent fasting. Actually, many experts agree that if you practice intermittent fasting but then overeat during your meal times, you are actually defeating the purpose of the practice. Rather, in order to really reap the benefits of intermittent fasting, the idea is to eat the right foods that will hold you over during your non-eating periods.

"IF works via calorie restriction," nutrition expert Dr. Mike Roussell, Ph.D. said in his report. "So if you fast for 24 hours but then eat twice the amount of food that you normally would during the subsequent 24 hours then the fast is essentially pointless." This is why the quality of what you eat during your meal times is so important.

The most important food groups to include when practicing intermittent fasting are animal proteins, vegetables, berries, and whole grains. "If you are intermittently fasting make sure you eating a full and satisfying meal filled with nutritious grains, vegetables and lean proteins," said Lyuda Bouzinova, an ACE-certified personal trainer and co-founder of Mission Lean.

"The goal is to get all of your nutrition from fewer meals so don't waste the space on your plate by filling it up with things that won't add anything beneficial to your body's biome," she said.

There is an ideal meal for someone intermittent fasting. "A plate of wild rice with some roasted salmon or baked cod prepared with delicious veggies and olive oil and add some avocado for extra creaminess," Bouzinova said.

"You will get tons of nutrition, feel satiated at the end of the meal, and will feel strong and energized when you wake up the next morning."

"There are no specifications or restrictions about what type or how much food to eat while following intermittent fasting," says Lauren Harris-Pincus, MS, RDN, author of The Protein-Packed Breakfast Club. But "the benefits [of IF] are not likely to accompany consistent meals of Big Macs," says Mary Purdy, MS, RDN, chair of Dietitians in Integrative and Functional Medicine.

Both Pincus and Purdy agree that a well-balanced diet is the key to losing weight, maintaining energy levels, and sticking with the diet. "Anyone attempting to lose weight should focus on nutrient-dense foods, like fruits, veggies, whole grains, nuts, beans, seeds, as well as dairy and lean proteins," Pincus says. Purdy adds, "My recommendations would not be very different from foods that I might normally suggest for improved health—high-fiber, unprocessed, whole foods that offer variety and flavor." To make it more clearer, I have highlighted and explain below some of the best food for intermittent fasting. In other words, eat plenty of the below foods and you won't end up in a hungry rage while fasting.

1. Water

Even though you aren't eating, it's important to stay hydrated for so many reasons, like the health of basically every major organ in your body. The amount of water that any one person should drink varies, but you want your urine to be a pale yellow color at all times. Dark yellow urine indicates dehydration, which can cause headaches, fatigue, and lightheadedness. Couple that with limited food, and it could be a recipe for disaster. If the thought of plain water doesn't excite you, add a squeeze of lemon juice, a few mint leaves, or cucumber slices to your water.

2. Avocado

It may seem counterintuitive to eat the highest calorie fruit while trying to lose weight, but the monounsaturated fat in avocado is extremely satiating. A study even found that adding a half of an avocado to your lunch may keep you full for hours longer than if you didn't eat the green gem.

3. Fish

There's a reason the Dietary Guidelines suggests eating at least eight ounces of fish per week. Not only is it rich in healthy fats and protein, it also contains ample amounts of vitamin D. And if you're only eating a limited amount of food throughout the day, don't you want one that delivers more nutrient-bang for your buck? Not to mention that limiting your calorie intake may mess with your cognition, and fish is often considered a "brain food."

4. Cruciferous Veggies

Foods like broccoli, Brussels sprouts, and cauliflower are all full of the f-word—fiber. When you're eating erratically, it's crucial to eat fiber-rich foods that will keep you regular and prevent constipation. Fiber also has the ability to make you feel full, which is something you may want if you can't eat again for 16 hours. Woof.

5. Potatoes

Repeat after me: Not all white foods are bad. Case in point: Studies have found potatoes to be one of the most satiating foods around. Another study found that eating potatoes as part of a healthy diet could help with weight loss. Sorry, French fries and potato chips don't count.

5. Beans and Legumes

Your favorite addition to chili may be your best friend on the IF lifestyle. Food, specifically carbs, supplies energy for activity. While we're not telling you to carbo-load, it definitely would not hurt to throw some low-calorie carbs, like beans and legumes, into your eating plan. Plus, foods like chickpeas, black beans, peas, and lentils have been shown to decrease body weight, even without calorie restriction.

6. Probiotics

You know what the little critters in your gut like the most? Consistency and diversity. That means they aren't happy when they're hungry. And when your gut isn't happy, you may experience some irritating side effects, like constipation. To counteract this unpleasantness, add probiotic-rich foods, like kefir, kombucha or kraut, to your diet. The Farmhouse

Culture Gut Shots are perfect for any 500-calorie days since each 1.5-ounce shot is brimming with live probiotics (10 billion CFUs) for just 10 calories.

7. Berries

Your favorite smoothie addition is ripe with vital nutrients. Strawberries are a great source of immune-boosting vitamin C, with more than 100 percent of the daily value in one cup. And that's not even the best part—a recent study found that people who consumed a diet rich in flavonoids, like those in blueberries and strawberries, had smaller increases in BMI over a 14-year period than those who did not eat berries.

8. Eggs

One large egg has six grams of protein and cooks up in minutes. Getting as much protein as possible is important for keeping full and building muscle. One study found that men who ate an egg breakfast instead of a bagel were less hungry and ate less throughout the day. In other words, when you're looking for something to do during your fasting period, why not hard-boil some eggs?

9. Nuts

They may be higher in calories than many other snacks, but nuts contain something that most junk food doesn't—good fat. Research suggests that polyunsaturated fat in walnuts can actually alter the physiological markers for hunger and satiety.

And if you're worried about calories, don't be! A 2012 study found that a one-ounce serving of almonds (about 23 nuts) has 20 percent fewer calories than listed on the label. Basically, the chewing process does not completely break down the almond cell walls, leaving a portion of the nut intact and unabsorbed during digestion.

10. Whole Grains

Being on a diet and eating carbs seem like they belong in two different buckets, but not always! Whole grains are rich in fiber and protein, so eating a little goes a long way in keeping you full. Plus, a new study suggests that eating whole grains instead of refined grains may actually rev up your metabolism. So go ahead and eat your whole grains and venture out of your comfort zone to try farro, bulgur, spelt, kamut, amaranth, millet, sorghum, or freekeh.

What can I drink during fasting?

The theory behind intermittent fasting is that your body stores fat for later use, allowing you to skip meals for up to 24 hours, sometimes longer. Even while you're not eating, there are some no- or low-calorie drinks are recommended for a fast. Always talk with your doctor before beginning a fast to be sure it is safe for you.

Coffee & Tea

I recommends drinking tea while fasting because it contains few calories and won't derail your weight loss. This means you cannot add sugar, cream or milk to your tea; drink it plain. You may also use artificial sweeteners if you prefer your tea sweetened. Both hot and cold tea are acceptable.

You also can drink coffee during intermittent fasting, but it must be black — no sugar, milk or cream, which contain calories. Use artificial sweeteners for flavor if you like. Avoid the coffee drinks in coffee shops, because most contain some type of syrup, milk product or sugary add-in.

Water

According to Maggie Moon, MS, RDN, author of The MIND Diet, intermittent fasting takes many forms, but most allow water. In fact, avoiding water for extended periods of time can be dangerous. "It is important to stay hydrated even when fasting," Moon says. "Dehydration can lead to unclear thinking, mood changes, constipation and kidney stones."

If there is some food intake involved during intermittent fasting (e.g. some plans call for around 500 calories per day on calorie restricted days), then Moon recommends about 9 cups of water for women and 12 for men.

But when food intake is restricted during intermittent fasting, more of your hydration will come from plain old water. General recommendations for daily water intake from all food and beverage sources are about 11 cups of water for women, and about 16 cups for men. According to the Centers for Disease Control and Prevention (CDC), most people can stay hydrated by simply letting thirst be their guide. For longer fasts, drink juice to keep up your strength.

Although, juice is not calorie-free and would not fit in with your intermittent fasting program. However, according to Moon, nutrients during fasting

are important. "I know "fasting" sounds like you aren't eating or drinking anything, but actually, the studies on intermittent fasting often includes some calories on "fasting days," she says.

Her recommendation is that one hundred percent juice is one way to provide energy and nutrients during fasting, but it needs to be integrated into a low-calorie plan. From that perspective, high-water, low-calorie foods may be more satisfying as it gives the fasting person a greater volume of food per calorie.

Other Low-Calorie Li□uids

Fruit-infused water is hydrating and may keep the palate more interested on fasting days. One of Moon's favorites is water infused with strawberries, oranges, and mint. She also recommends unsweetened almond milk, which tends to be low in calories and is fortified with calcium and vitamin D.

Finally, warm, savory clear broths can help make a low-calorie meal feel more satisfying. For example, vegetable, chicken or beef broth.

Recipes for intermittent fasting may include;

Bacon, Egg & Asparagus Keto Bowl
Low-Carb Veggie Full English Breakfast Bowl

Low-Carb Chocolate Coconut Smoothie
Healthy Salmon & Tabbouleh Low-Carb Bowl
Healthy Low-Carb Lemon & Lime Cooler
Low-Carb All Day Mexican Bowl
Easy Pork Chops With Asparagus and Hollandaise
Anti Keto Flu Nourish Bowl
Keto Portobello Mushroom Mini Pizzas
Sugar-Free Lemon Granita
Healthy Low-Carb Caprese Omelet
Healthy Blueberry & Lemon Electrolyte Drink
Healthy 5-Minute Tuna Salad
Keto Superfood All Day Breakfast Skillet
Healthy Sesame Crusted Salmon with Coconut Cauli-Rice
Healthy Chicken, Bacon & Spinach Salad
Low-Carb Green Veggie Soup with Halloumi Croutons
Healthy Keto Electrolyte Smoothie Bowls
Keto Salmon, Kale & Poached Egg Bowl

How To Prepare For Intermittent Fasting?

If anyone is thinking about starting intermittent fasting, it is best to first switch to a low-carbohydrate, high-healthy fat diet for three weeks. This will allow the body to become accustomed to using fat rather than glucose as a source of energy. That means getting rid of all sugars, grains (bread, cookies, pastries, pasta, rice), legumes, and refined vegetable oils. This will minimize most side effects associated with fasting.

Start with a shorter fast of 16 hours, for example, from dinner (8 pm) until lunch (12 pm) the next day. You can eat normally between 12 pm and 8 pm, and you can eat either two or three meals. Once you feel comfortable with it, you can extend the fast to 18, 20 hours.

For shorter fasts, you can do it everyday, continuously. For more extended fasts, such as 24-36 hours, you can do it 1-3 times a week, alternating between fasting and normal eating days.

There is no single fasting regimen that is correct. The key is to choose one that works best for you. Some people achieve results with shorter fasts, others may need longer fasts. Some people do a classic water-only fast which will discuss later, others do a tea and coffee fast, still others a bone broth fast. No matter what you do, it is very important to stay hydrated and monitor yourself. If you feel ill at any point, you should stop immediately. You can be hungry, but you should not feel sick.

Who is Intermittent Fasting Good For?

As you can see, there are a plethora of different methods of varying difficulty when it comes to intermittent fasting, so it's not necessarily a one-size-fits-all diet. Considering the benefits and risks, IF may be best for people who enjoy a wide range of foods and who struggle with diets that restrict certain types of food groups or macronutrients. With IF, the focus isn't on the Quality or even the Quantity of food you're eating, rather just the time frame that you're eating in. So, if you want to keep pasta, chocolate, and wine on the table while staying "on your diet," it may be a palatable option.

IF may also be helpful for those who tend to have digestive problems at night time as bumping up the last meal of the day before bed may help prevent heartburn, acid reflux, and other digestive woes.

While early research suggests that fasting may have some benefits on blood sugar control, individuals with insulin-dependent diabetes should likely avoid radical fasting regimens. Enjoying regular, healthy meals can help prevent blood sugar spikes and dips that can be life-threatening for diabetics if not controlled. It may also not be ideal for amateur or professional athletes who depend on perfectly timed fuel before and after activity for athletic performance and recovery.

It is important to note that drinking certain low or no-calorie drinks is usually allowed when practicing intermittent fasting and it's really important to always stay hydrated. Intermittent fasting is not an easy habit to keep up with, but getting dehydrated will make it even harder. Dehydration can cause headaches, fatigue, and dizziness which would derail your intermittent fasting pretty □uickly. Most intermittent fasting plans allow for unsweetened coffee or tea, water, and broths, so make sure whatever type of plan you choose you know which li□uids are allowed and you fill up on those. One thing is definitely a must, though. "Avoiding refined starches, added sugars, trans fats, and processed meats still hold true!"

CHAPTER 4

BENEFITS OF INTERMITTENT FASTING EXPLAINED

The benefits of intermittent fasting are vast. Fasting gets a bad rap, but as explained before, there is real science behind the techni□ue of fasting, in particular, intermittent fasting. Many people think that someone who is fasting has an eating disorder, but nothing could be farther from the truth.

The truth is that in today's society, we eat far too much and too often. Our bodies are very precise mechanisms that, allowed to run properly, will take care of us far beyond our imagination. The problem lies with the fact that historically, for thousands and thousands of years, we were a species with little food resources and we worked long and hard each and every day for the morsels we did get. Today, we have a plethora of food, most of it very fattening, and sedentary lifestyles. This both contributes to obesity and disease.

Fasting intermittently can eliminate many problems caused from overeating and sitting around all day instead of out hunting and gathering. The fact is that we have not evolved enough to be able to handle all the calories that we ingest on a daily basis, our bodies still operate as if we were hunter and gatherers. Not until the 20th century did most people have food at the ready, so 100 years is not even close to enough time to change how our body operates.

The biggest benefit of intermittent fasting is simplicity. Some few years ago, in an interview with Vanity Fair, President Obama described an interesting strategy he uses to make his life simpler. "You'll see I wear only gray or blue suits," he said. "I'm trying to pare down decisions. I don't want to make decisions about what I'm eating or wearing. Because I have too many other decisions to make."

What President Obama is referring to is a concept called "decision fatigue" and it can drastically impact your ability to make decisions throughout the day. For the President, simplifying his clothing choices is a way to make life simpler and improve his decision making abilities. For me, intermittent fasting provides the same benefit. Eliminating breakfast and not thinking about food until a particular set time each day has allowed me to reduce the number of decisions

I make in the morning, thus reducing decision fatigue and increasing the willpower I have for the rest of the day. That means I have more energy to put toward doing work that is important to me.

One of the best ways to find happiness and success in life is to strip away the unnecessary things and focus only on what is needed. With intermittent fasting, I have been able to increase strength, reduce body fat, and maintain good health while spending less time eating each day. If you can get the same results by making life simpler and only eating twice per day, why would you make life more complex by eating three, four, or five times per day?

The health benefits of intermittent fasting Explained

1)   Intermittent Fasting Changes The Function of Cells, Genes, and Hormones.

When you don't eat for a while, several things happen in your body. For example, your body initiates important cellular repair processes and changes hormone levels to make stored body fat more accessible.

Here are some of the changes that occur in your body during fasting:

Insulin levels: Blood levels of insulin drop significantly, which facilitates fat burning.

Human growth hormone: The blood levels of growth hormone may increase as much as 5-fold. Higher levels of this hormone facilitate fat burning and muscle gain, and have numerous other benefits.

Cellular repair: The body induces important cellular repair processes, such as removing waste material from cells.

Gene expression: There are beneficial changes in several genes and molecules related to longevity and protection against disease.

Many of the benefits of intermittent fasting are related to these changes in hormones, gene expression and function of cells. When you fast, insulin levels drop and human growth hormone increases. Your cells also initiate important cellular repair processes and change which genes they express.

2. Intermittent Fasting Can Help You Lose Weight and Belly Fat

Many of those who try intermittent fasting are doing it in order to lose weight. Generally speaking, intermittent fasting will make you eat fewer meals. Unless if you compensate by eating much more during the other meals, you will end up taking in fewer calories.

Additionally, intermittent fasting enhances hormone function to facilitate weight loss. Lower insulin levels, higher growth hormone levels and increased amounts of norepinephrine (noradrenaline) all increase the breakdown of body fat and facilitate its use for energy.

For this reason, short-term fasting actually increases your metabolic rate by 3.6-14%, helping you burn even more calories. In other words, intermittent fasting works on both sides of the calorie e☐uation. It boosts your metabolic rate (increases calories out) and reduces the amount of food you eat (reduces calories in).

According to a 2014 review of the scientific literature, intermittent fasting can cause weight loss of 3-8% over 3-24 weeks. This is a huge amount. The people also lost 4-7% of their waist circumference, which indicates that they lost lots of belly fat, the harmful fat in the abdominal cavity that causes disease.

One review study also showed that intermittent fasting caused less muscle loss than continuous calorie restriction. All things considered, intermittent fasting can be an incredibly powerful weight loss tool. More details will be discuss in subse□uent chapter on how Intermittent Fasting Can Help You Lose Weight.

Intermittent fasting helps you eat fewer calories, while boosting metabolism slightly. It is a very effective tool to lose weight and belly fat.

3. Intermittent Fasting Can Reduce Insulin Resistance, Lowering Your Risk of Type 2 Diabetes

Type 2 diabetes has become incredibly common in recent decades. Its main feature is high blood sugar levels in the context of insulin resistance. Anything that reduces insulin resistance should help lower blood sugar levels and protect against type 2 diabetes.

Interestingly, intermittent fasting has been shown to have major benefits for insulin resistance and lead to an impressive reduction in blood sugar levels. In human studies on intermittent fasting, fasting blood sugar has been reduced by 3-6%, while fasting insulin has been reduced by 20-31%.

One study in diabetic rats also showed that intermittent fasting protected against kidney damage, one of the most severe complications of diabetes. What this implies is that intermittent fasting may be highly protective for people who are at risk of developing type 2 diabetes.

However, there may be some differences between genders. One study in women showed that blood sugar control actually worsened after a 22-day long intermittent fasting protocol. Intermittent fasting can reduce insulin resistance and lower blood sugar levels, at least in men.

4. Intermittent Fasting Can Reduce Oxidative Stress and Inflammation in The Body

Oxidative stress is one of the steps towards aging and many chronic diseases. It involves unstable molecules called free radicals, which react with other important molecules (like protein and DNA) and damage them. Several studies show that intermittent fasting may enhance the body's resistance to oxidative stress.

Additionally, studies show that intermittent fasting can help fight inflammation, another key driver of all sorts of common diseases. Intermittent fasting can reduce oxidative damage and inflammation in the body. This should have benefits against aging and development of numerous diseases.

5. Intermittent Fasting May be Beneficial For Heart Health

Heart disease is currently the world's biggest killer. It is known that various health markers (so-called "risk factors") are associated with either an increased or decreased risk of heart disease. Intermittent fasting has been shown to improve numerous different risk factors, including blood pressure, total and LDL cholesterol, blood triglycerides, inflammatory markers and blood sugar levels.

However, a lot of this is based on animal studies. The effects on heart health need to be studied a lot further in humans. Overall, studies show that intermittent fasting can improve numerous risk factors for heart disease such as blood pressure, cholesterol levels, triglycerides and inflammatory markers.

6. Intermittent Fasting Induces Various Cellular Repair Processes

When we fast, the cells in the body initiate a cellular "waste removal" process called autophagy.

This involves the cells breaking down and metabolizing broken and dysfunctional proteins that build up inside cells over time. Increased autophagy may provide protection against several diseases, including cancer, and Alzheimer's disease.

7. Intermittent Fasting May Help Prevent Cancer

Cancer is a terrible disease, characterized by uncontrolled growth of cells. Fasting has been shown to have several beneficial effects on metabolism that may lead to reduced risk of cancer.

Although human studies are needed, promising evidence from animal studies indicates that intermittent fasting may help prevent cancer. There is also some evidence on human cancer patients, showing that fasting reduced various side effects of chemotherapy.

8. Intermittent Fasting is Good For Your Brain

What is good for the body is often good for the brain as well. Intermittent fasting improves various metabolic features known to be important for brain health.

This includes reduced oxidative stress, reduced inflammation and a reduction in blood sugar levels and insulin resistance.

Several studies in rats have shown that intermittent fasting may increase the growth of new nerve cells, which should have benefits for brain function. It also increases levels of a brain hormone called brain-derived neurotrophic factor (BDNF), a deficiency of which has been implicated in depression and various other brain problems. Animal studies have also shown that intermittent fasting protects against brain damage due to strokes.

Intermittent fasting may have important benefits for brain health. It may increase growth of new neurons and protect the brain from damage.

9. Intermittent Fasting May Help Prevent Alzheimer's Disease

Alzheimer's disease is the world's most common neurodegenerative disease. There is no cure available for Alzheimer's, so preventing it from showing up in the first place is critical.

A study in rats shows that intermittent fasting may delay the onset of Alzheimer's disease or reduce its severity. In a series of case reports, a lifestyle intervention that included daily short-term fasts was able to significantly improve Alzheimer's symptoms in 9 out of 10 patients.

Animal studies also suggest that fasting may protect against other neurodegenerative diseases, including Parkinson's and Huntington's disease.

10. Intermittent Fasting May Extend Your Lifespan, Helping You Live Longer

One of the most exciting applications of intermittent fasting may be its ability to extend lifespan. Studies in rats has shown that intermittent fasting extends lifespan in a similar way as continuous calorie restriction.

In some of these studies, the effects were quite dramatic. In one of them, rats that fasted every other day lived 83% longer than rats who weren't fasted.

Although this is far from being proven in humans, intermittent fasting has become very popular among the anti-aging crowd.

Given the known benefits for metabolism and all sorts of health markers, it makes sense that intermittent fasting could help you live a longer and healthier life.

What are Some of the Concerns of Intermittent Fasting?

1. It could cause infertility in some people

We know that adequate caloric and nutrient intake is essential for reproductive health, particularly because amenorrhea (loss of menstrual cycle) is directly linked to under eating and low body weight. While we don't have any large human trials specific to IF, it's quite possible that the restrictive nature of the diet can interfere with nature doing its thing. In fact, one animal study found that an IF regimen interfered with the fertility of rats.

2. It could impair athletic performance.

Getting the most out of your workout really comes down to carefully timed fuel, and restricting calories for long periods of the day can definitely get in the way. Not only can it leave you too sluggish to really push the pedal to the medal, but if your workout isn't timed perfectly during your "feasting" phase, you could be missing out on a really important window for muscle growth and glycogen replenishment. The result is that you might actually start breaking down metabolism-boosting muscle, not building it.

3. It seems hard to stick to in the long run.

Like most diets, IF can be really hard to stick with in the long run. One study actually compared IF to daily caloric restriction and found that the dropout rate was significantly higher among fasters than calorie-cutters. Interestingly, this study also suggested that the individuals assigned to the fasting group gradually just ended up cutting calories over time, suggesting that this may just be a more natural way to eat.

4. It could cause disordered eating.

While it's not officially documented, I can attest that it's very easy for people in the "diet mindset" to overdo their "feast" phase. In other words, if you're given free rein to eat whatever you want for a short few hours and you're hungry when you get there, it's not unreasonable to assume you're going to face plant into the first thing you see. Hello, office donuts! Not only will this negate any weight-loss benefits, but it's also possible it can lead to some dangerous disorderly binging behaviors over time.

No one will have the same experience as you — with intermittent fasting or with anything else — and that's why you have to experiment on your own. It might be easier to cite a study or follow the advice of some diet guru, but the only way to get results is to test, adjust, and repeat.

As you may have noticed, it's appealing to think that fasting might be an ancient survival mechanism that triggers healing processes in the body, as many fasting researchers suggest, but that doesn't mean all forms of fasting are the same or that they have the same health effects. Many will vary from person to person, and you should always consult your doctor before trying any severe dietary changes.

In his new book, "The Longevity Diet," Longo cautions against using the term "intermittent fasting" too broadly. We know various forms of fasts — like eating only during certain hours, restricting eating one or two days a week — are associated with health benefits. But we don't know that all these health benefits are the same for all fasts. But even so, many of these intermittent-fasting regimens are considered relatively safe for a healthy person. So if they appeal, they could be worth a shot as they may come with a host of health benefits.

CHAPTER 5

INTERMITTENT FASTING SYSTEM AS A WEIGHT LOSS TOOL

Individuals uses intermittent fasting to lose weight fast. In studies done by the NIH, there was reported weight loss with over 84% of participants — no matter which method of fasting they chose (alternate day fasting, the 8/16 method, or another approach). Science has shown intermittent fasting to be an efficient weight loss tool, sometimes more than simply cutting calories. In one study, intermittent fasting was shown to be as effective as continuous calorie restriction in fighting obesity.

Intermittent fasting has been shown to increase fat loss while maintaining lean muscle mass. In one four-week study, researchers concluded that a fasting diet resulted in greater weight loss — while maintaining muscle mass — than participants following a low-calorie diet. This happened even though the total calorie intake over the four weeks was similar in both groups.

When following a ketogenic diet, fasting can help you enter ketosis, the desired metabolic state for weight loss and fat burning, more quickly. The longer you remain in a healthy state of ketosis, the better. Following a ketogenic diet while practicing intermittent fasting can help keep you in ketosis, even after breaking a fast.

When you go for an extended period of time without eating, your body changes the way that it produces hormones and enzymes, which can be beneficial for fat loss. These are the main fasting benefits and how they achieve those benefits.

Hormones form the basis of metabolic functions including the rate at which you burn fat. Growth hormone is produced by your body and promotes the breakdown of fat in the body to provide energy. When you fast for a period of time, your body starts to increase its growth hormone production. Also, fasting works to decrease the amount of insulin present in the bloodstream, ensuring that your body burns fat instead of storing it.

A short term fast that lasts 12-72 hours increases the metabolism and adrenaline levels, causing you to increase the amount of calories burned. Additionally, people who fast also achieve greater energy through increased adrenaline, helping them to not feel tired even though they are not receiving calories generally. Although you may feel as fasting should result in decreased energy, the body compensates for this, ensuring a high calorie burning regime.

Most people who eat every 3-5 hours primarily burn sugar instead of fat. Fasting for longer periods shifts your metabolism to burning fat. By the end of a 24-hour fast day, your body has used up glycogen stores in the first few hours and has spent approximately 18 of those hours burning through fat stores in the body. For anyone who is regularly active, but still struggles with fat loss, intermittent fasting can help to increase fat loss without having to ramp up a workout regime or drastically alter a diet plan.

Simple guide on how to Lose Fat With Intermittent Fasting

I will be using the 8:16 intermittent fasting plan which to me, is the simplest form of intermittent fasting. In intermittent fasting you simply divide the day into two phases:

Phase 1: Feeding phase of 8 hours
Phase 2: Fasting phase of 16 hours

By doing that, you will be unable to eat more than 2-3 solid meals a day and the 16 hour fasting phase enables you to lose fat. This is a very effective approach for a skinny-fat guy, because to lose fat you have to eat less calories than you burn! In my opinion, the easiest and most enjoyable way to lose fat, is by implementing intermittent fasting into your lifestyle since it is very SIMPLE. As an added benefit, a lot of people experience that they are very productive during their fasting phase, since they are not spending their mornings on preparing breakfast and eating.

If you are a student, intermittent fasting could look similar to this:

- 07 AM: Wake up and drink a cup of coffee.
- 12 AM-08 PM: Feeding Phase
- 08 PM-12 AM: Fasting Phase

As you can see above, it is actually very simple: instead of breakfast you drink a nice cup of coffee (without sugar) and you stay productive until noon to avoid eating. When your 8-hour feeding phase starts, you eat 2-3 solid meals that fuel your workout. After your last meal you can unwind and enjoy your evening until you go to bed. I have experienced success with this approach, even though I eat what I want with each of my meals, as long as the majority of my food intake is healthy.

Therefore... if you implement intermittent fasting into your life style you can forget everything about:

- Eating small unfulfilling meals every 2-3 hours
- Waking up early to prepare breakfast
- Experiencing insulin spikes in the afternoon
- Counting calories

Proof That Intermittent Fasting and Bodybuilding Work Together

Intermittent fasting and bodybuilding can work for you if your goal is to build muscle and to get lean and here are 3 reasons why.

1. Recent studies have shown that it is in actual fact total macros and the total amount of daily calories that account for muscle growth and not the amount of meals and the timing of them. Essentially what this is saying is that as long as you get the re□uired amount of calories in the 24 hour period it doesn't matter when you get them. So as long as you get your re□uired amount of calories (a surplus of your TDEE is needed in combination with a

progressive training routine) in your eating window you will gain muscle.

2. One facet of intermittent fasting bodybuilding that people complain about is the amount of food and calories that need to be consumed within the eaten window. Although you most likely will need to adjust if you are currently eating 6-8 small meals a day, over a period of a couple of weeks you stomach will adjust to eating larger meals. Some people found it very difficult to eat large meals in the beginning but within a week or so they can adjust and have no problems putting away large amounts of food in one sitting. Take your time with the adjustment period and don't expect to be able to switch over night.

3. Remember, like everything else intermittent fasting isn't an exact science and if you need to extend our eating window from say an eight hour eating window to a nine hour window to accommodate your total calories and meal re□uirements, that's fine go ahead and do so. Like any program, it's important to find what works for you. Intermittent fasting, bodybuilding and building muscle can work together and the beauty of it is if you find that sweet spot that works for you you'll get the benefits of intermittent fasting while maintaining or building your physique to a bodybuilding level.

One of the most famous bodybuilders of his generation Sergio Nubret was a strong advocate of intermittent fasting way back before it was popular. Sergio Nubret had a fantastic physi□ue and whether or not he built that body using steroids is not the question here, what his nutritional methods were are.

Amazing Body

Sergio Nubret was famous not only for having an impeccable physique; he was also famous for his style of nutrition. He ate like a lion in the African wild. No, he didn't go around chasing zebra and antelope. He simply ate one gargantuan meal each day and the remainder of the day he fasted. Essentially, what he was practicing was intermittent fasting. He had a window where he would eat his meal and a window where he would not.

Can you emulate him using intermittent fasting?

If he built such an impressive physi□ue using a one meal a day method, surely you can tap into your genetic potential for bodybuilding using an intermittent fasting model of 2-3 or even 4 meals a day. It's □uite easy to fit 3-4 meals a day into an eight hour eating period. For example, if your eating window starts at 12pm, you could have your first meal at 12pm, your second at 3pm your third at 6pm and your fourth at 8pm. It's pretty much the same as eating every 2-3 hours it just means you get to have bigger portions (always a good thing).

Calorie Surplus for muscle building

At the end of the day, whether or not you can build muscle doesn't come down to how many meals you have, it comes down to whether or not you're in a calorie surplus, if you're training progressively and are in a calorie surplus you will build muscle so this suggests that intermittent fasting and bodybuilding can work for you. It worked for Sergio Nubret and he ate only one meal a day. There are a lot of other success stories available from the likes of Brad Pilon, John Berardi, Martin Berkhan and the Hodgetwins that show significant muscle growth while intermittent fasting.

Iike I will emphasize again, just like everything it may or may not be the best option for you, what's important is that you find out if that is the case and don't dismiss it until you have at least experiment with it. The benefits of intermittent fasting are pretty amazing and combined with a proper training program and nutrition you can build muscle to bodybuilding standards.

Tips on how to Succeed With an Intermittent Fasting Protocol for weight loss

Here are 5 tips to help you get started on an effective intermittent fasting system for weight loss.

Don't make your fast too long or too short

An ideal fast length for weight-loss and health benefits is between 16 and 24 hours depending on age, experience and exact goals. Any less than this won't really give you the results you want (remember you are already fasting for 10-12 hours overnight) and any longer than this is simply unnecessary and can be harder to adapt to.

Increase your water intake when fasting

Intermittent fasting will also help to cleanse your system and let your body work more efficiently. In order to help this process, you should increase your water intake. The best way to do this is have a glass/bottle of water with you at all times so that you can sip regularly.

Break your fast with a healthy meal

The first thing you eat after a fast should be a healthy meal. Apart from the obvious benefits of eating healthy food, this also leaves less space for eating junk. Given that you might only have 8 hours to eat your daily food, filling up on the good stuff first is always a good option.

Time your food around your workouts

I will not end this section without saying that working out should be part of any healthy eating plan. The centre piece of your training efforts should be weight-training or bodyweight training. Try to eat most of your food in the period immediately after your workout. In this way, your body will be more likely to use these calories to rebuild and repair rather than be stocked as fat.

Don't sweat the details

One of the real benefits of intermittent fasting is that it is not necessary to count calories or grams of macronutrients. This can be a pain and makes diets difficult to stick to. Follow principles and the details will take care of themselves.

Overall, intermittent fasting can be a great tool to lose body fat and body weight. It can also be a mentally-positive alternative to those who struggle with calorie counting and portion control.

The key with fasting — as with any weight loss plan — is to find what works for you. Focus on healthy foods in between fasts, and remind yourself that you are taking control of your body, health, and future.

Why I Favor Intermittent Fasting Over Calorie Restriction

Intermittent fasting also has a number of added benefits over strict calorie restriction. For starters, it's a lot easier to comply with, and compliance is everything. The calorie restriction route is also extremely dependent on high quality nutrition — you want to sacrifice calories without sacrificing any important micronutrients — and this can be another hurdle for many who are unfamiliar with nutrition and what actually constitutes a healthy diet.

You also want to avoid the counting calories and calorie restriction fallacies. Most people fail to appreciate that there are many intricate biochemical dynamics that occur that are unaccounted for when you just count "calories in and calories out." While animals like rats can achieve a 40 percent increase in longevity through lifelong calorie restriction, such a great effect is not seen in humans, and there are good reasons for that.

"There is a good evolutionary explanation for the difference in the calorie restriction response when comparing short-lived and long-lived species: famines are seasonal, and a season is a large fraction of a mouse lifespan but a small fraction of a human life span. Thus only the mouse evolves a relatively large plasticity of life span in response to food scarcity."

In terms of calorie restriction and weight, humans also tend to have an innate resistance to excessive weight loss, even in the face of severe calorie restriction. Dr. Ancel Keys demonstrated this in the mid-1940s when he designed an experiment to investigate the impact of starvation on human beings.

Thirty-six young healthy male volunteers were placed on a 24-week calorie-restricted diet of about 1,600 calories per day. They also had to walk for about 45 minutes a day. But instead of resulting in continuous weight loss, at 24 weeks their weight had stabilized, and no more weight loss could be elicited even when he reduced calorie intake down to 1,000 or less per day.

The drawbacks were clear. The men became obsessed with food to the exclusion of everything else in their life, and when the calorie restriction ended, they all over-reacted. Within a few weeks, they regained all of the lost weight plus about 10 percent more. Other studies have come to similar conclusions. So starvation-type diets may not be ideal for the average person. Your body will tend to shut down various processes in order to survive. For example, by reducing thyroid function, your body will not burn as many calories.

All of this may seem hopelessly contradictory. On the one hand, calorie restriction promotes beneficial biological changes that tend to extend life; on the other, there are built in mechanisms that when triggered by chronic calorie restriction can trigger other health problems. These are complex issues, and any extreme measure is likely to cause more problems than it solves.

The best we can do is come up with some general guidelines that replicate ancestral patterns. In my view, daily intermittent fasting and avoiding eating for a number of hours has many advantages over general calorie restriction and other radical diets, while providing many of the same benefits with a minimum of risk.

To Lose Fat You Need to Retrain Your Body to Burn Fat for Fuel

When you consistently eat every few hours and never miss a meal, your body becomes very inefficient at burning fat as a fuel, and this is where the trouble starts. It's important to recognize that, with few exceptions, you cannot burn body fat if you have other fuel available, and if you're supplying your body with carbohydrates every few hours, your body has no need to dive into your fat stores. When you apply intermittent fasting, you not only avoid this but also will typically decrease your food costs and increase your health.

Eating fewer meals and timing those meals to occur closer together, is one of the most effective strategies I've found to trigger your body to more effectively burn fat for fuel, and normalize your insulin and leptin sensitivity. If you're not insulin resistant, intermittent fasting is not as crucial, but may still be beneficial.

If you're among the minority of Americans who do not struggle with insulin resistance, then my general recommendation is to simply avoid eating at least three hours before bedtime. That automatically allows you to "fast" for at least 11 hours or longer depending on if and when you eat breakfast.

Equally important is the recommendation to EAT REAL FOOD when you do eat, meaning food in the most natural form you can find, ideally whole organic produce, and pasture-raised when it comes to meats and animal products like diary and eggs. To that, I would add avoiding sitting, engaging in non-exercise movement throughout the day, and getting regular exercise. Exercise will not produce significant weight loss without addressing your diet, but when done in combination it can be significantly beneficial.

CHAPTER 6

INTERMITTENT FASTING FOR WOMEN- IS INTERMITTENT FASTING SAFE FOR WOMEN TOO?

For women who are interested in weight loss, intermittent fasting may seem like a great choice, but many people want to know, should women fast? Is intermittent fasting effective for women? Everyone comes into this world imbued with attributes, characteristics, and predilections that are uni□uely theirs. We're all humans, but we're a diverse bunch, and that makes it interesting. And though it also makes giving cookie cutter health advice impossible, I just take that as an opportunity to stand out from the crowd and provide actionable advice that genuinely helps real people.

A perfect example is biological sex. Anyone who's lived with the opposite sex, been married, or had kids of different sexes knows that males and females are different—on average.

There's a ton of overlap, don't get me wrong.

We all need fat, protein, and carbohydrates. We all have the same requirements for sustenance and wellness. We all breathe oxygen, get stronger and fitter when we work out, use the same neurotransmitters, and produce the same hormones. The biological basics are identical, It's the details that differ and matter.

Fasting As Hormetic Stressor and the Influence of Biological Sex

Men and women both need to enter a "fasted" state in order to burn body fat. This should go without saying, but regularly undergoing periods where you're not inserting calories into your mouth is an absolute requirement for weight loss and basic health, no matter your sex.

These periods are called "fasted states," and they begin as soon as you stop processing the energy from your meal. An "intermittent" fast is an extended period of not eating done for the express purpose of weight loss and other health benefits.

By definition, a fast is a hormetic stressor—a stressful input (no food) that in the right dose triggers an adaptive response that makes us stronger and healthier. Fasting triggers Nrf2, the "hormetic pathway" also triggered by other hormetic stressors like exercise, polyphenols, and radiation. Nrf2 initiates a series of defensive and adaptive mechanisms that help you respond to the stress and buttress your body against future stressors. But with too large a dose, a hormetic stressor can become a plain old stressor—one that overwhelms our defenses and harms us.

Making matters more complicated, the size of a hormetic dose is relative. What's hormetic for me might be stressful for you. Many different variables affect how much of a hormetic stressor a person can tolerate. With fasting, perhaps the most important variable to consider is your biological sex. This really does make intuitive sense.

Biology cares most about your fertility. Can you reproduce? Can you produce healthy offspring that survive to do the same? These things come first. And from that perspective, a woman's situation is more precarious than a man's. You have a finite number of eggs, or "chances." Men have an almost infinite supply of sperm.

When you are preparing to get pregnant, your body needs extra nutrients to build up a reserve and "prime the pump." When you are pregnant, the growing baby needs a reliable and constant stream of nutrients for almost a year. After a man gets someone pregnant, his biological involvement with the growing baby is done. What or when he eats has no impact on the survival of the growing baby.

After you've given birth, the growing newborn needs breastmilk. To make that milk requires additional calories and extra doses of specific nutrients. Modern technology allows us to skip nursing and go straight to the bottle, but your body doesn't "know" that.

It all points to women being more finely attuned to caloric deficits. For example, women's levels of ghrelin, the hunger hormone, are □uicker to rise after meals. This isn't just relevant for parents or parents-to-be. Even if you're not interesting in getting pregnant and having kids, or you have children and aren't planning on any more, the ability to do so is strongly connected to your health. Reproductive health is health. As far as your body's concerned, having kids is the primary goal and you need to be ready to do it as long as you're able.

While intermittent fasting does seem to offer some promising health benefits, it may not be for everyone — especially depending on whether you're male or female. And as it stands now, there's more research being done on intermittent fasting for rats than for humans.

It seems that whether or not intermittent fasting will work for you comes down to human biology. While shorter periods of fasting are generally considered safe for most people, some of the extended fasting times associated with intermittent fasting can be disastrous for a woman's hormones — causing things such as reproductive issues and early menopause — and may worsen other pre-existing health conditions.

Some of the general benefits of intermittent fasting for women may include:

Sustainable weight loss
An increase in lean muscle mass
More energy
An increase in cell stress response (which could increase resistance against some diseases)
A reduction in oxidative stress and inflammation
Improvement around insulin sensitivity in overweight women
Increased production of neurotrophic growth factor (which could relieve depression, boost cognitive function, and protect against neurodegenerative diseases, such as Alzheimer's)

Now, here's the tricky part. Although intermittent fasting may have its benefits, women are naturally sensitive to signs of starvation, so intermittent fasting for women is a whole different beast.

When the female body senses it's headed towards famine, it will increase the production of the hunger hormones, ghrelin and leptin, which signal to the body that you're hungry and need to eat. Additionally, if there's not enough food for you to survive, your body is going to shutdown the system that would allow you to create another human. This is the body's natural way of protecting a potential pregnancy, even if you're not actually pregnant or trying to conceive.

It's not that you're intentionally imposing a famine upon yourself — but your body doesn't know that. It doesn't know the difference between true starvation and intermittent fasting, which is why it defaults to this protective mechanism.

Therefore, some of the cons due to hormonal imbalances brought on by intermittent fasting may also lead to:

Irregular periods and amenorrhea (complete loss of period)
Metabolic stress

Shrinking of the ovaries
Anxiety and depression
Fertility issues
Difficulty sleeping

Since all of your hormones are so deeply interconnected, when one hormone is thrown off balance, the rest are also negatively impacted. It's like a domino effect. As the "messengers" that regulate nearly every function in your body — from energy production, to digestion, metabolism, and blood pressure — you don't want to disrupt their natural rhythm.

With all of these drawbacks, you may be wondering: could you (and would you still want to) practice intermittent fasting as a female? If you take a more relaxed approach, the answer is YES. When done within a briefer timeframe, intermittent fasting can still help you reach your weight loss goals and provide the other health benefits previously mentioned, without messing up your hormones.

The Best Intermittent Fasting Methods for Women

8/16 Method

This method is one of the best ways to ease into intermittent fasting without shocking your body or aggravating your hormones. It doesn't require you to fast every day, only a few days per week, spaced throughout the week. For example, Monday, Wednesday and Friday.

Fasting Window: 12-16 hours
Eating Window: 8-12 hours
Safe for Women: Yes

16/8 Method

The 16/8 method is another brief intermittent fasting routine that's used specifically to target body fat and improve lean muscle mass (a.k.a. your gains!).

Fasting Window: 16 hours
Eating Window: 8 hours
Safe for Women: Yes

24 Hour Protocol (a.k.a. "Eat-Stop-Eat")

The 24-hour protocol, also known as "eat-stop-eat" requires you to do a 24-hour fast, once or twice a week. You can choose the time you start fasting. Some people prefer to fast from 8pm to 8pm the following day, or begin their fast after breakfast.

Fasting Window: 24 hours
Eating Window: 0

Safe for Women: Yes, when done a maximum of 2 times per week.

The 5:2 Diet

The 5:2 diet, also known as the "Fast Diet," involves restricting calories two days a week to 500 calories per day (with two 250 calorie meals), while eating normally for the other five days. For example, you might eat all of your regular meals Saturday through Wednesday, and eat 500 calories per day on Thursdays and Fridays. Since it doesn't completely restrict food on the fasting days, it may also be an effective way to ease into fasting without shocking your system. This Fasting system is considered safe for men and women.

Fasting Window: No fasting window, just calorie restriction to 500 calories per day for 2 fasting days per week
Eating Window: Assume regular caloric intake 5 days per week
Safe for Women:

When Should You Avoid Intermittent Fasting as a woman?

Intermittent fasting isn't a good fit for everyone. You should not consider intermittent fasting if you are:

Pregnant
Nursing
Under chronic stress
Have a previous history of disordered eating, such as bulimia or anorexia
Struggle with sleep disorders, or have difficulty sleeping

Additionally, intermittent fasting is meant to complement a healthy diet and lifestyle — not act as a way to remedy five days of eating nutritionally-bankrupt foods, such as refined sugar, processed foods and fast foods.

Intermittent Fasting For Women Over 50

Obviously our bodies and our metabolism changes when we hit menopause. One of the biggest changes that women over 50 experience is that they have a slower metabolism and they start to put on weight. Fasting may be a good way to reverse and prevent this weight gain though. Studies have shown that this fasting pattern helps to regulate appetite and people who follow it regularly do not experience the same cravings that others do. If you're over 50 and trying to adjust to your slower metabolism, intermittent fasting can help you to avoid eating too much on a daily basis.

When you reach 50, your body also starts to develop some chronic diseases like high cholesterol and high blood pressure. Intermittent fasting has been shown to decrease both cholesterol and blood pressure, even without a great deal of weight loss. If you've started to notice your numbers rising at the doctor's office each year, you may be able to bring them back down with fasting, even without losing much weight.

Some Thoughts For Women Who Want to Fast

Don't fast unless you have a good reason. Good reasons include:

Having significant amounts of fat to lose.
Your oncologist giving you the go-ahead to try using it to improve the effects of chemotherapy.
Your neurologist giving you the go-ahead to try using it to improve brain function in the face of cognitive decline or dementia.

Bad reasons include:

Keeping the pregnancy weight at bay.
Going from 15% body fat to 12%.
To boost your 5x weekly CrossFit sessions.

Intermittent fasting for women has some beneficial effects. What makes it especially important for women who are trying to lose weight is that women have a much higher fat proportion in their bodies. When trying to lose weight, the body primarily burns through carbohydrate stores with the first 6 hours and then starts to burn fat. Women who are following a healthy diet and exercise plan may be struggling with stubborn fat, but fasting is a realistic solution to this. Although, intermittent fasting may not be a great idea for every woman. Anyone with a specific health condition or who tends to be hypoglycemic should consult with a doctor. However, this new dietary trend has specific benefits for women who naturally store more fat in their bodies and may have trouble getting rid of these fat stores.

Intermittent fasting may work amazingly well for some people, and terribly for others. Most importantly, if you do decide to give intermittent fasting a try, be sure to listen to your body's feedback. Easing into intermittent fasting by starting with shorter fasting windows can help with initial symptoms of hunger and discomfort. But if it becomes too uncomfortable, be honest with yourself, accept it, and move on. At the end of the day, nothing can have a greater impact on your health than a diet rich in real, whole foods, and a lifestyle that prioritizes your physical, mental, and emotional well-being.

CHAPTER 7

HOW ABOUT LONG FASTING OR WATER FASTING - A COMPARISON WITH INTERMITTENT FASTING

On the whole, Intermittent fasting is a powerful tool for improving health, jump-starting weight loss, or beating cravings, and there's plenty of medical literature to back up its usefulness. But what about longer fasts (more than a day or two)? If intermittent fasting is good, will a longer fast be even better?

Long-term fasting can take several different forms. The most extreme is a "dry fast," consuming nothing at all (food or water). This is definitely not advisable, as it's very dangerous to go for more than a day or so without drinking. Water fasting means drinking only water, but consuming no calories during the fast. Another technique is juice fasting, or consuming only fruit and vegetable juices. Some people also fast on broth, or extremely low-calorie protein mixes.

Juice fasting and bone broth fasting aren't truly fasts since they do involve some intake of calories and nutrients. And protein fasts can be downright dangerous, since humans just weren't built to live on protein with no accompanying fat. This chapter focuses on water fasting: the comparison with intermittent fasting, the benefits, the drawbacks, and precautions to take if you do decide to start a longer fast.

What is water long fasting?

There are several different ways to detox your body that can involve expensive programs and methods, but the most simple, inexpensive approach just might be the best way of all. Water fasting to detoxify your body will shift the body's focus away from digesting foods that you are not eating while fasting and work at restoring a balance once again. When you are not eating solid foods for a few days and drinking only water, the body's system will begin a detoxification process, eliminating built up waste that has been accumulating within the body.

Given the chance, your body knows how to maintain itself and clean itself out when the focus is taken off of ingesting food for a short time. When looking for water fasting weight loss you should know that detoxification phase, the body's system will work hard at getting rid of the toxic build up and accumulation of waste that the body has in it's system.

Fasting will help kick in a regeneration cycle within your body. This is the body's natural way of cleaning house. Many people will water fast a couple of times a year to help the body regulate itself better. It's like giving your system a tune up.

The body will normally get it's energy from glucose. This is a natural form of sugar that is in many of the foods we eat. We converts this glucose from the food or liver, which stores this, turning the glucose into glycogen. When we start to fast, this sugar source gets used within the first day of fasting. When we continue to fast past the first day, the body will derive it's fuel supply from our fat reserve cells. When looking for water fasting weight loss you should know that within the third day of a water fast, our bodies are running almost exclusively on our stored fat cells with a minimum amount of the body's muscle being consumed.

Water Fasting for Weight Loss - Good or Bad?

Water fasting is, exactly that! Just water-no solid food, juices, coffee, tea or milk. Are there any benefits to such drastic measures? And does it work?

Well a surgeon may re☐uest this just 24 hours before an operation or some other medical procedure, or it may be part of a religious ritual. Maybe some people are happy to just drink pure water for a short length of time thinking this will flush out all the build of toxins in the system and restore a natural balance. Water fasting weight loss can occur over a period of time. If you are considering fasting for long periods it is always wise to consult with your GP first and foremost giving your reasons as to why you want to engage in this other than other forms of fasting.

A one day fast, once a week, once a month appears to be the most common time limit but even then you must prepare yourself for this. A few days before engaging on a water fasting weight loss system, spend a couple of days drinking fruit juices and eating very little so that your body starts to get used to not having solid food. Water is one of the main important elements in your diet, without this it can lead to all sorts of problems with kidney function, circulatory and digestive systems. When you water fast, it gives the body an opportunity to cleanse itself. How much water you drink is personal to yourself, but on average drink a large glass full of pure water, with nothing added, every few hours or so depending on your size and how active you are. Any clean water is ade□uate, filtered tap water and bottled water is fine provided it is just pure water-nothing added. If your urine is pale yellow then you know you have an ade□uate intake. If you are running to the toilet every few minutes then that is too much, and if your urine is a dark yellow-then you will need to drink more as you will dehydrate.

Water fasting for weight loss can work and will definitely show results but you have to be very strong willed and determined to water fast for many days. It has been claimed that to show any real results then you have to water fast for at least 21 days to a maximum of 40 which, in my opinion, is a very daunting and drastic measure! However if you have medical problems i.e. heart problems, hyperglycemia, or see a GP regularly for other complaints then have a consultation and get monitored by a health professional first. Dizziness and a feeling of weakness are common ailments during water fasting weight loss diet.

There is no doubt that water fasting can help you shed pounds but it also slows down your metabolism, as your body expects solid food, and once you start to slowly introduce food back into your system then your body will hold onto this food storing it as fat and the weight you have lost could be regained. So perhaps the water fasting weight loss diet should be part of a healthier lifestyle, to include a balanced diet with regular exercise, to obtain a good overall feeling of well-being with the added bonus of weight loss.

Other Benefits of long or water fasting

In addition to weight loss, water fasting also promotes autophagy, which is like a "spring cleaning" for your cells. Since your body is essentially eating itself, it has a chance to get rid of any junk or waste material that may have built up, and repair the damage of oxidative stress. This is one of the biggest benefits of fasting even for people who are already at a healthy weight, since it has powerful anti-aging and muscle-building properties.

One study also found that an extended fast (10 days on average) was beneficial to patients with hypertension, also noting that even though the patients didn't embark on the fast to lose weight, all of them did – average weight loss was around 15 pounds. Longer term fasting (up to 5 days) may also have some benefits for chemotherapy patients.

Another benefit of extended fasting is purely mental: for many fasters, it's a way to "re-set" their relationship with food, break free from patterns of emotional eating, or start fresh at the end of the fast. Fasting is part of many religious and spiritual practices because of its value for meditation and mindfulness. Bear in mind that this doesn't happen automatically: it requires a high level of self-awareness and effort on the part of the faster. It's a very useful tool, but it's not a miracle cure.

Dangers and Drawbacks of long or water fasting

The ultimate risk of long fasting, of course, is death by starvation; this doesn't usually happen to people fasting for medical reasons, but taking anything to extremes is perilous. In Ireland in 1981, for example, 10 political prisoners starved themselves to death in a hunger strike against the British government, fasting between 46 and 73 days before they died.

Even fasts of a few weeks or less can have dangerous consequences. Fasting puts two different types of stress on your heart. First, it cannibalizes cardiac muscle for fuel. The human body does everything it can to conserve muscle during a fast, but inevitably some muscle will be sacrificed at the beginning of the fast. After a few days, the body switches over to using fat, but researchers have discovered that protein (muscle) utilization actually increases again later on, even though fat stores are still available. This protein includes the muscle in your heart: weaken this too much, and heart failure will result.

Strict water fasting is also a risk for heart failure because during a fast, the body's intracellular stores of minerals vital for cardiac function, like magnesium and potassium, are depleted, even though serum levels remain normal. The results of this cardiac muscle loss and mineral deprivation can be tragic. During the 1950s and 60s, fasting was used as an experimental treatment for obesity, and several patients died (many from heart failure). Other reports of people dying during long fasts include more cases of heart failure. More recently, in 2010, a woman in Florida died after 21 days of fasting.

Other fasters die of infectious diseases that they simply don't have the energy to fight off without adequate nutrition. In 1978, for example, a man named William Carlton died of pneumonia at a fasting center after fasting for 29 days in an attempt to cure his ulcerative colitis. He was 49 years old, and in normal health other than the colitis. Worldwide, infectious diseases are actually the most common cause of death among starving people, because an immune system weakened by malnutrition tends to give in before heart problems start to show. This is particularly common among children who go on (or are forced to go on) long fasts.

Of course, many people also fast safely, but it's worth noting that long fasting isn't a risk-free experiment. Less serious drawbacks also include intense mood swings, low energy, and irritability. Long fasting may lowers blood pressure, so you may feel weak, dizzy, or nauseous during the fast. It raises levels of the stress hormones norepinephrine and cortisol, probably an adaptation to give you more energy for finding food, but not beneficial for optimum health.

Another potential downside of long-term fasting is the rate of detox. Fat is your body's storage organ for everything, including any toxins that may have accumulated over the years. When you lose weight, all these toxins have to be removed through your bloodstream, which can be extremely uncomfortable. During fasting, these symptoms are even more pronounced, since the rate of fat burning is so rapid – many people feel nauseous, sick, or otherwise unwell.

Detox is sometimes a necessary evil, but when you're thinking about the potential dangers of long-term fasting, make sure not to get taken in by fanatical advocates who claim that everything is just another detox symptom. Sometimes it's actually a symptom of a bigger problem, not just detox, and even rapid detox can be unhealthy in itself.

There's also a darker side to the mental health benefits of long fasting. For eating disordered people, fasting can □uickly turn into another form of abuse (punishment for eating too much or anything "wrong.") Because fasting is often accompanied by a strange kind of energy, it's possible to get addicted to it, and ignore physical danger in pursuit of that "fasting high." This is just as dangerous as any other form of chronic malnutrition and starvation.

Water or Long Fasts vs. Intermittent fasting

With any dietary intervention, you want to get the most gain for the least amount of pain. Especially considering that the benefits of intermittent fasting (as opposed to longer fasts) are so well attested, it's worth a look to see if shorter fasts aren't a better idea overall.

So are long or short fasts superior? The answer is that it depends on why you're fasting. You can get the physical benefits of longer fasts just as easily from intermittent fasting, or even from not fasting at all. Ketosis, for example, doesn't require any calorie restriction, only carbohydrate restriction. Since a ketogenic diet includes all the vitamins and nutrients your body needs to keep functioning, it's much less dangerous and easier to just eat ketogenic meals than to enter ketosis by fasting.

Autophagy is also achievable through intermittent fasting just as easily as longer fasts. Autophagy begins when liver glycogen is depleted, around 12-16 hours into a fast. The rate of autophagy peaks there, and then drops after about 2 days. If your goal is a "spring cleaning" for your cells, intermittent fasting may be even more effective, since you spend more time in the "early fasting" period when autophagy is at its peak.

Long fasts also lose points for the social aspect – it's easy to plan family meals around an 8-hour feeding window, but much more difficult to stay engaged in a healthy social life if you're avoiding food altogether.

Intermittent fasting also reduces many of the drawbacks of long fast. There's typically no loss of lean tissue (muscle), since people who IF eat plenty of protein, just at different times. Intermittent fasting allows you to keep working out, while exercising during long fasts will just cause more muscle loss. There's much less risk of malnutrition, heart failure, and infectious complications with intermittent fasting – from a physical perspective, it's hard to see how anyone would prefer an extended water fast.

On the other hand, there are some emotional and psychological benefits of longer fasts that intermittent fasting just doesn't provide. A 2 or 3 week fast can be a springboard for a radical change in dietary habits – fasters report that abstaining from food completely gave them a valuable chance to re-evaluate their eating habits. For example, even emotional eating of ketogenic or otherwise healthy foods doesn't break you out of the cycle of eating to deal with uncomfortable feelings. A total fast forces you to find other ways of handling these emotions. This can make a fast very difficult, but also very rewarding for people who can stick it out.

On the whole, intermittent fasting is superior for physical health (the same gain with less risk), but longer fasting may be superior for emotional, psychological, or spiritual reasons.

Precautions for long-term fasters

If you do decide to embark on a long fast, some common-sense precautions can prevent prevent a disappointing failure – or worse, a trip to the emergency room. Some people simply shouldn't practice extended fasts, period:

Young children are still growing rapidly and need ade□uate nutrition at every stage to make sure their bodies develop properly

Very elderly people often don't have the physical resources to fast safely.

People who are seriously ill, or people with chronic heart or kidney conditions, should not fast since their bodies may not be able to withstand the stress of fasting.

Women who are pregnant, or trying to get pregnant, should eat plenty of nutrient-dense food, because a well-fed state is essential for healthy reproduction.

If you're not in any of these groups, make sure to do your own research and have a plan beforehand. Read up on other people's experiences with long fasts, so you understand what you're getting into. Think about your physical and emotional relationship with food – what do you think will be the difficulties of fasting for you, and how will you overcome them? Are there any specific issues that you want to meditate on or work through while you're fasting?

A useful fasting plan should also include a plan for dealing with other people during your fast. Unless you live alone, chances are good that someone will notice and be concerned. How will you reassure them that you're not anorexic or starving yourself? What if you have to participate in a business lunch or another work meeting involving food?

Also, make a backup plan while you're well-fed and healthy for what you'll do if the fast isn't going well. During a long fast, it's normal to experience crazy emotional highs and lows; this can prevent you from making a rational decision about whether or not you want to continue. Write down your criteria for what will make you stop the fast ("I will stop fasting if my blood pressure drops below ________________" or "I will stop fasting if I lose __________ pounds" or whatever it might be for you) and stick to them during your fast.

An even better option is to find someone to supervise your fast. If at all possible, it's wise to fast under the care of a doctor, but this isn't always an option, since most mainstream doctors have a knee-jerk negative reaction towards lomg-term fasting. Even a close friend with no medical training can help provide some valuable perspective on how the fast is going. Fasting centers are another option, but these also aren't without their problems: some of the fasting experts who run them have been implicated in very sketchy practices, and it's crucial to do a lot of research before entrusting yourself to them.

During your fast, make sure to drink plenty of water to avoid dehydration, and take supplemental electrolytes: sodium, potassium, calcium, phosphate, and magnesium. Your body needs these minerals to balance fluid levels, and supplementing also prevents one of the chief dangers of fasting: refeeding syndrome. Normally, you get those minerals from your food; since you're continuing to drink water without eating anything, you need them from an alternate source during your fast. You can buy "electrolyte water" (make sure you don't get sports drinks full of artificial flavorings, though), make your own with water, lemon, and a pinch of salt, or take supplements.

While you're in the midst of a fast, don't try to work out at all – this will just cause your body to lose more muscle than necessary. The closer you can get to bed rest, the better. Read journal, meditate, sleep, listen to music, or talk to people you love. Many people take time off work to concentrate on their fast. Keeping a slow-paced and thoughtful environment will help you really get the most of the psychological and spiritual benefits of fasting.

Water or Long-term fasting is definitely an intriguing idea. Humans certainly have the ability to endure long periods of famine, but that doesn't mean it's healthy. So far, there's some substantial evidence showing benefits for weight loss, but whether this weight loss is actually sustainable in the long term remains to be proven. And in most cases, you can get all the physical benefits of long-term fasting from intermittent fasting, without all the attendant risks of completely abstaining from food for several weeks at a time. So for purely physical health reasons, longer fasts aren't great because they have increased dangers without any increased benefits.

For the vast majority of people, it's a much better idea to use intermittent fasting or alternate-day fasting (24 hours of feeding followed by 24 hours of fasting) and perhaps a ketogenic diet to reap the physical benefits of food restriction, without the very real dangers of longer fasts. For mental health and spiritual practice, on the other hand, longer fasts do have some advantages over intermittent fasting. Whether the benefits outweigh the risks is a decision everyone has to make individually – don't take the dangers lightly, and make sure to do your own research before you make your choice.

CHAPTER 8

MYTHS ABOUT INTERMITTENT FASTING, MEALS AND WEIGHT LOSS

As with all popular fitness or health trends, there are many myths out there about intermittent fasting that aren't quite right or simply aren't true at all.

A few of the most common myths about intermittent fasting are:

Your Body Enters Starvation Mode
Skipping Breakfast = Weight Gain
You Should Eat Small Meals Frequently
Fasting Slows Down Your Metabolism
You'll Get Too Hungry
You'll Lose Muscle
Your Brain Needs Fuel
You'll Gain The Weight Back
You'll Overeat Between Fasting Periods
You Won't Get Enough Nutrients
Its just plain unhealthy

The body eats itself, or it stores each and everything you eat because it thinks food is no longer available."

1. Your Body Will Enter Starvation Mode If You Fast

Even if you've never heard of intermittent fasting before, you've probably been warned against skipping meals because your body will go into "starvation mode." According to this idea, not eating makes your body think it's starving, which shuts your body's metabolic processes down. Your body is saving energy because it's not sure when it will get nutrients again, which prevents you from burning fat.

While it's true that your body does change when you are fasting, evidence shows that short-term fasting actually increases your body's metabolic functions. Starvation mode is a real thing, but it takes long periods of actual starvation – not short periods of fasting intermittently.

2. Skipping Breakfast Causes Weight Gain

We've all been told since we were children that breakfast is the most important meal of the day, right? A popular claim that opposes intermittent fasting is that if you don't eat breakfast, you'll gain weight.

Skipping breakfast will make you hungrier throughout the day, so you're more likely to gorge on food later, the claims say.

When you're a child or a teenager, breakfast is definitely important – it helps you do better in school because you're not concentrating on being hungry. But as long as you are health conscious with the rest of the meals you eat later in the day after skipping breakfast, you should have no trouble skipping breakfast while fasting.

3. You Should Eat Small Meals Frequently

Eating small meals throughout the day instead of eating three large meals is supposed to help lose weight, keep weight off and avoid the effects of feeling hungry. There is no evidence that frequent meals boost your metabolism or reduce hunger. Therefore, it can't be proven to have any effect on weight loss. Some people personally may feel that eating small meals a few times a day instead of three large meals (or instead of intermittent fasting) is better for them.

If you are likely to make unhealthy choices when you're hungry, this might be a good method for you. But if you make healthy food choices every day, there is no reason to eat multiple small meals many times a day.

4. Fasting Slows Down The Metabolism
Many people associate intermittent fasting with crash diets, so the claims go that when you don't give your body the food it needs, your metabolism will slow down and adapt to survive on less calories.

But because you are eating and fasting intermittently, instead of going without eating at all, your body is getting the calories it needs – just at a different time than it's used to.

In that same vein, many people believe eating more fre□uently will boost your metabolism. But numerous studies show that there is no difference in calories burned if you eat more fre□uently.

5. You'll Get Too Hungry

Many people believe that fasting intermittently causes your body to get too hungry, and in response, you will feel compelled to overeat between fasting periods.

After beginning intermittent fasting, you will feel hungry, but your body adapts to the change and your feelings of hunger decrease over time. There's also a chance your feelings of hunger throughout the day aren't true hunger pains but a mental focus on the lack of food.

You know it's lunchtime, so you feel hungry. Or your body is thirsty, so you feel hungry. Your body isn't crying out for food, but you feed it anyway.

6. You'll Lose Muscle

Some people do believe that fasting will lead to starvation mode, which will cause your body to begin burning muscle and using it for fuel. This does happen with all sorts of diet plans and patterns, but there's no evidence that intermittent fasting causes it more than others. It's also more often associated with crash dieting than intermittent fasting.

Intermittent fasting doesn't involve cutting out exercise or not giving your body the calories that it needs to function – just changing when you eat.

7. Your Brain Needs Fuel

Because studies have shown that children and teenagers function better at school after getting a balanced breakfast, the idea has formed that not eating will lead to your brain not getting the fuel it needs to function. The claims say that if you are fasting, your brain can't function properly, and you will experience poor concentration and memory loss.

Not exactly. The brain does need glucose (blood sugar) to operate, but it can also get this from proteins. Your brain will not stop functioning if you don't eat every few hours.

Even during long-term fasting or starvation diets (which I don't recommend, by the way!) the body can produce what it needs for proper brain functioning.

8. You'll Gain The Weight Back

Again, people tend to associate intermittent fasting and other popular health trends with crash diets. Many people who participate in these crash diets lose a lot of weight but gain it all back after the diet is over.

However, it's not because of the diet itself.

Rather, diets often do not teach people how to make better decisions or build better habits – they only help to lose weight in the short term. People who are intermittently fasting could still gain back any weight that they lose if they don't follow a maintenance plan in between fasting periods.

9. You'll Overeat Between Fasting Periods

Some people claim that intermittent fasting will cause you to overeat between fasting periods, so you will actually gain weight or maintain your weight instead of losing it. This may be partly true. People do tend to eat a little bit more than they would've normally after fasting.

But studies show that most people who are intermittently fasting do not eat such an excessive amount after a fast that they cancel out the benefits of the fasting. It also has to do with the choices you make between fasting periods.

If you are eating slightly more than usual but still making healthy choices, there is a huge difference than if you are turning to processed foods or fattening choices.

10. You Won't Get Enough Nutrients

If you fast intermittently and then make unhealthy choices during the eating periods, then this myth may hold true. But all intermittent fast diets re□uire the participant to eat healthy during the eating periods, both to ensure the body gets what it needs and also to prevent gaining back any weight that is lost.

11. Its just plainly unhealthy

We spend a lot of time feasting in this country—Thanksgiving, Halloween, Christmas, birthdays, weddings, BBQs in the summer, and that is totally ok. Good food should be celebrated with people we love and the momentous occasions that go with it.

What we need to be pairing with feasting—and what has been largely forgotten about— is how to counter act the feasting with all the benefits of fasting. Let's put it this way—if improving insulin resistance, lowering insulin levels, lowering cortisol, improving brain fog, and supercharging energy levels, brain power, effortless weight loss tool, and increasing growth hormone to make you look and feel younger is wrong... I don't want to be right.

12. The body eats itself, or it stores each and everything you eat because it thinks food is no longer available."

There is a degree of truth to this as it applies to losing weight. Your body is not stupid or suicidal, if you have body fat to burn your body will burn it before it starts to consume lean tissue. Also, this myth takes a very short sighted look at how your body works. When you look at weight loss you should not measure it day to day, but rather, at a minimum, week to week.

If you look at results week to week you have enough data to actually draw a conclusion. Let's say for the sake of argument that on Monday your body does freak out and end up storing more of what you eat as fat than what it normally would. When your body gets done freaking out things will go back to normal and everything will even out. So even if it does freak out on Monday, by Friday or Saturday it will have evened out. So if you do go through periods where you don't consume as much you MIGHT store more of the little amount you do eat, but if that does happen it will all even out over time, AND your body will still break down and consume body fat if it needs to. "Starvation mode", as it is commonly talked about in the fitness industry, is largely a myth.

The only time you will go into actual starvation mode is if you are completely out of excess body fat or if you are unable to access your body's fat storage to use it as fuel. If you go up to a starving person and give him a cheeseburger, because he is actually starving, his body will store everything it can and he will only defecate a small portion of it. It is important to understand that, in a healthy person, PROLONGED FASTING LEADING TO KETOSIS is what happens when a person doesn't have an ample supply of calories in the bloodstream, muscle cells, or liver to meet its needs and starts breaking down stored body fat for energy, STARVING is what happens AFTER you run out of excess body fat and your body is forced to start breaking down lean tissue for energy to survive. This fact cannot be over-emphasized.

Think about it this way, our caveman predecessors went through fre□uent periods of not having any food available. If they were unable to eat for a day or two do you think their body would freak out and keep hold of their stored fat and start burning their muscle tissue and organ tissue for energy? No, if it did they would have all died and none of us would be here today. In times where you don't have food, your body will try to protect your lean tissue and use your fat tissue as fuel, after all that is what it is there for.

If you have more body fat than the typical American then you can last even longer. A morbidly obese person weighing over 300 lbs. can go several months surviving off of body fat until it is all depleted and the person needs to consume lean tissue.

Myths about meal debunked

Breakfast is the most important meal of the day

We have been told over and over again that we need to eat, almost immediately after we wake up.

That getting the right breakfast is starting the day off right. The truth is, we have been in a fasted state while sleeping, and it perfectly alright, and dare I say, encouraged, for you to eat when AND ONLY WHEN you feel hungry. Not just because you woke up, but because you are legit hungry. Drink a tall glass of water when you wake up—you'll likely find your hunger goes away. Feelings of hunger and thirst are almost identical. You'll probably find your hunger was masking as thirst. The most important meal of the day is not breakfast. Rather, when you break your fast.

Skipping Breakfast Will Make You Fat

As explained above, there is an ongoing myth that there is something "special" about breakfast. Also, People believe that breakfast skipping leads to excessive hunger, cravings, and weight gain. Although many observational studies have found statistical links between breakfast skipping and overweight/obesity, this may be explained by the fact that the stereotypical breakfast skipper is less health-conscious overall.

Interestingly, this matter was recently settled in a randomized controlled trial, which is the gold standard of science.

This study was published in 2014 and compared eating breakfast vs skipping breakfast in 283 overweight and obese adults. After a 16-week study period, there was no difference in weight between groups. This study shows that it doesn't make any difference for weight loss whether you eat or don't eat breakfast, although there may be some individual variability.

However, there are some studies showing that children and teenagers who eat breakfast tend to perform better at school. There are also studies on people who have succeeded with losing weight in the long term, showing that they tend to eat breakfast.

This is one of those things that varies between individuals. Breakfast is beneficial for some people, but not others. It is not essential and there is nothing "magical" about it. Eating breakfast can have benefits for many people, but it is not essential and will not necessarily make you fat. Controlled trials do not show any difference between eating and skipping breakfast for the purpose of weight loss.

Eating Frequently Boosts Your Metabolism

"Eat many, small meals to stoke the metabolic flame." Many people believe that eating more meals leads to increased metabolic rate, so that your body burns more calories overall.

It is true that the body expends a certain amount of energy digesting and assimilating the nutrients in a meal. This is termed the thermic effect of food (TEF), and amounts to about 20-30% of calories for protein, 5-10% for carbs and 0-3% for fat calories. On average, the thermic effect of food is somewhere around 10% of the total calorie intake. However, what matters here is the total amount of calories consumed, not how many meals you eat. Eating six 500-calorie meals has the exact same effect as eating three 1000-calorie meals. Given an average thermic effect of 10%, it is 300 calories in both cases.

This is supported by numerous feeding studies in humans, showing that increasing or decreasing meal frequency has no effect on total calories burned. There is no difference in calories burned if you eat more frequently. Total calorie intake and macronutrient breakdown is what counts.

Eating Frequently Helps Reduce Hunger

Some people believe that snacking helps prevent cravings and excessive hunger. Interestingly, several studies have looked at this, and the evidence is mixed. Although some studies suggest that more frequent meals lead to reduced hunger, other studies find no effects, and yet others show increased hunger levels.

One study that compared 3 high-protein meals to 6 high-protein meals found that 3 meals were actually better for reducing hunger. That being said, this may depend on the individual. If snacking helps you experience fewer cravings and makes you less likely to binge, then it is probably a good idea.

However, there is no evidence that snacking or eating more often reduces hunger for everyone. Different strokes for different folks. There is no consistent evidence that eating more often reduces overall hunger or calorie intake. Some studies even show that smaller, more freuent meals increase hunger.

The Brain Needs a Constant Supply of Glucose

Some people believe that if we don't eat carbs every few hours, that our brains will stop functioning. This is based on the belief that the brain can only use glucose (blood sugar) for fuel.

However, what is often left out of the discussion is that the body can easily produce the glucose it needs via a process called gluconeogenesis.

This may not even be needed in most cases, because your body has stored glycogen (glucose) in the liver that it can use to supply the brain with energy for many hours.

As noted earlier, even during long-term fasting, starvation or a very low-carbohydrate diet, the body can produce ketone bodies from dietary fats. Ketone bodies can provide energy for part of the brain, reducing its glucose re□uirement significantly.

So, during a long fast, the brain can easily sustain itself using ketone bodies and glucose produced from proteins and fats. It also makes no sense from an evolutionary perspective that we shouldn't be able to survive without a constant source of carbohydrate. If that were true, then humans would have become extinct a long time ago.

However, some people do report that they feel hypoglycemic when they don't eat for a while. If this applies to you, then perhaps you should stick to a higher meal fre□uency, or at least ask your doctor before changing things.

Overall, the body can produce glucose to supply the brain with energy, even during long-term fasts or starvation. Part of the brain can also use ketone bodies for energy.

Eating Often and Snacking is Good For Health

It is simply not "natural" for the body to be constantly in the fed state.

When humans were evolving, we had to endure periods of scarcity from time to time. As mentioned before, there is evidence that short-term fasting induces a cellular repair process called autophagy, where the cells use old and dysfunctional proteins for energy.

Autophagy may help protect against aging and diseases like Alzheimer's disease, and may even reduce the risk of cancer. The truth is that fasting from time to time has all sorts of benefits for metabolic health.

There are also some studies suggesting that snacking, and eating very often, can have negative effects on health and raise your risk of disease. For example, one study found that, coupled with a high-calorie intake, a diet with more frequent meals caused a greater increase in liver fat, indicating that snacking may raise the risk of fatty liver disease.

There are also some observational studies showing that people who eat more often have a much higher risk of colorectal cancer. It is a myth that snacking is inherently good for health. Some studies show that snacking is harmful and others show that fasting from time to time has major health benefits.

Myths about weight and fat loss debunked

There are five nutrition myths that can and do sabotage many of our weight loss goals. Here is what I know so far:

1 - Good weight loss programs need to be complicated with special charts and graphs and calorie calorie cycling. Limiting what to eat and when to eat based on your specific metabolic type / blood type / birthstone / horoscope sign.

The fact is the simpler the program the better the results will be. The more restrictive the diet, the more likely you will fail. A bad weight loss plan will be complicated and hard to follow practically guaranteeing failure. That is the first reason why I will recommend intermittent fasting.

2: "If you're dieting you need to focus on eating protein because protein builds muscle and burns fat."

Protein, carbohydrates, and fat are the three primary macro-nutrients (source of calories) and they don't cancel each other out like a game of rock, paper, scissors. Consuming protein can support fat loss in three ways. The first way is that protein can support muscle growth (if the necessary calories are there and if muscle growth is stimulated through work or damage) and since muscle cells re□uire more calories than fat cells to survive the more muscle you have the more calories you burn overall.

The second benefit protein can offer fat loss is by extending digestion time. Fats and carbohydrates normally exit the stomach in under an hour once consumed, but by eating protein with the fat and carbohydrates, you can offer the body something more time consuming to break down and it will be 3 to 4 hours until the last of that meal leaves the stomach. Where this CAN be of benefit is that by eating protein you can get your stomach to release food to your body over a longer period of time and this can keep your blood sugar from spiking and help it stay more level. More on this in Myth 3.

The third way is that protein is harder for your body to break down so it re□uires you to burn more energy to process it. I've heard claims that due to the increased amount of energy required to digest protein eating a large protein filled breakfast was the same as jogging 3 to 4 miles in terms of energy expenditure, but the problem with this is that while it does take more energy to process protein it doesn't necessarily e□uate to fat loss. What determines fat loss is how many calories you consume in a 24-hour period or a one week period vs. your total expenditure. Eating more protein can increase your TEF (explained in myth 3) and, when combined with the amounts of your BMR and AI (also explained in myth 3) can lead to an increase in fat loss, but it not the actual protein itself that is responsible for the burning of any extra fat that could possibly result.

One place where this myth comes from is a misguided notion of what protein is and does, and also there have been studies done that you could read as supporting this myth. Studies have looked at the weight loss of people who ate higher and lesser amounts of protein in their diet and most have found that the more protein people eat the more fat they tend to lose. The problem is that if you look at the studies closely you'll see that those eating more protein filled up on protein -rich food and as a result they ate far less carbohydrates and fat and consumed less calories total. It is the decrease in the consumption of carbohydrates, fat, and calories in general that lead to the weight loss.

The last thing I'll say about this is that there is nothing wrong with eating a high protein diet while trying to lose weight and there is evidence to suggest it may be a good idea. Did the increased protein consumption in the studies mentioned above make the participants feel fuller faster and make them feel fuller longer? Yes, it did. Is there evidence to suggest that eating more protein while trying to lose fat is a good idea? Yes, provided you eat less carbohydrates and fat leading to you consuming fewer calories than you need each day.

So protein can have an effect that supports your efforts to eat less, and protein CAN have an effect that supports your overall weight loss goals. Protein, however, in and of itself does not build muscle nor burn fat.

3: "To lose weight you need to eat 6 small meals a day to lose weight."

When people find out that I only eat one or two meals a day and I'm a firm believer in intermittent fasting people look at me like they're trying to figure out how I'm still alive. This is a good example of the fact that if you repeat something enough times people will start to regard it as true. We've already talked about the nonsense of "starvation mode" and the necessity of eating multiple small meals all day long to lose weight.

First, it should be mentioned that the studies that tested this method for weight loss defined a "meal" as anything consumed, li□uid or solid, that was over 45 calories. So the studies that looked at this method of numerous small meals didn't have people stop and eat a traditional meal 5 or 6 times a day. They would eat three traditional meals a day and have two or three meals that might have consisted of a small handful of nuts or even a low-calorie beverage. That being said let's look at the nuts and bolts of this theory as regard to weight loss.

If you eat a "meal" consisting of at least one exchange (for the purpose of this book let's say that exchange means "serving") of each protein, carbohydrates, and fat it will take 3 to 4 hours to leave your stomach, and if you repeat this every 3 to 4 hours your body will be digesting food all the waking hours of the day. By doing this you will achieve two benefits; firstly by having the food leave your stomach slowly you MIGHT prevent a spike in insulin levels and since insulin is a hormone that tells your body to store energy, by not having a spike you will have less of a signal to store the food you just ate. Lower insulin levels means less of the food you just ate will be stored as fat and it will either be burned for energy or passed through you and end up in the toilet.

The second benefit is that by doling out food slowly you will keep your blood sugar fairly level all day. If your blood sugar goes above 120 milligrams per deciliter you will have an insulin surge and if your blood sugar goes below 80 milligrams per deciliter you will feel hungry. So the thought is that by keeping your blood sugar between 80 to 120 milligrams per deciliter you will store less of what you eat and feel less hungry.

It sounds good, but is it good? We'll it isn't bad.

If you like eating this way then you should absolutely continue, but it just isn't necessary. The actual benefits of this type of diet are more behavioral than physiological. Many people find that by focusing on set pre-planned meals they think about eating less and find that they can stick to a diet better. People tend to find that since they are eating several times a day they are less hungry, but is that because their blood sugar is kept level or is because they're constantly eating? Is it both? There is nothing wrong with this but it just isn't the weight loss law the "experts" claim that it to be nor does it necessarily have the benefits they claim it does.

As we already know, the "experts" are wrong when they claim that if you don't eat several small meals a day you'll go into "starvation mode" and the world will end, but they also claim that eating this way boosts your metabolism. They say that your metabolism is like a furnace and you need to keep feeding the furnace to keep your metabolism going and burn calories. Is this true? Yes and no (but, in context, mostly no).

There is no end of things that are supposed to "boost your metabolism" so let's look at your metabolism a little deeper. Metabolism is the process where your body builds things and tears things down to keep you alive. How the term is used in the fitness industry is to mean the rate at which you burn calories. This is a very narrow definition of metabolism but it is the one that we will use.

In using this definition, there are three things that regulate how many calories you burn a day (again, assuming you are healthy). Those things are your basal metabolic rate (BMR), your activity index (AI), and the thermogenic effect of food (TEF). What this all means is that your body spends energy on only three things: 1.) running the bodily functions that keep you alive, 2.) making you move, and 3.) digesting the food you eat and processing it into energy.

Your basal metabolic rate (BMR) is how many calories it takes to do nothing more than run your body and keep you alive for 24 hours. If you were in a coma it is how many calories you'd burn in a day. It is not taking into account anything other than keeping you alive.

Your activity index (AI) is all the movements you make in a day. It is all the movements an average person makes just living, such as yawning and walking, plus any extra exercise like deliberate running, playing sports, or going to the gym. The thermogenic effect of food (TEF) is the energy it takes to digest and process everything you eat, and we've already talked about this a little when we discussed protein.

Those three elements make up your metabolism and determine how many calories you burn in a day. Most of the things that are supposed to boost your metabolism (like pills) merely make your heart beat faster and increase your AI. Eating more protein will slightly increase your TEF.

So where in this math does eating 6 meals a day speed anything up? Taking a set amount of food and consuming it in 6 meals versus just 3 doesn't affect your BMR and since it is the exact same amount of food it doesn't really affect your AI or TEF either.

The way they get away with saying that eating increases metabolism is because "truth-in-weight-loss police" don't exist, and because in a very small way it does. If you eat something your body has to digest it and it does take energy so you are metabolizing something and for those minutes your net energy expenditure does increase, but in a way that is not necessarily meaningful.

Your metabolism is going all day long and does not stop until you die. Since your body spends most of your energy on your BMR, just keeping you alive, the most meaningful way to increase or decrease it is to weigh more or less so it has more or less of you to keep alive.

This is also why eating less, consuming fewer calories, and controlling your insulin is the secret to losing weight. If you run on a treadmill for an hour and burn 300 calories you just spent an awful lot of energy, an hour of your time, and now your body might have 300 calories to makeup. But, if instead of going to the gym you look at what you eat in a day and decide to switch to diet soda and eat two fewer muffins during the day the small effort you just made could cut out 800 calories from your diet.

If you need 1500 calories a day to stay alive, you burned another 350 by moving all day long, and another 120 by digesting food that means you need 1950 calories for that day. If by cutting out the muffins and soda you only took in 1150 your body has to come up with the missing 800 calories because math is math. Since a pound of fat contains roughly 3500 calories, if you did that for 7 days you'd lose just over a pound and a half (assuming hormones don't get in the way, more on that later).

While very beneficial, exercise is not a very effective way to lose fat. You can go to the gym and kill yourself every day but until you eat less than what you need you won't really lose fat. The main benefit exercise has, in terms of weight loss, is in "body reshaping". Through exercise you can build muscles and develop a strong toned figure that fat loss can uncover.

One thing that should be mentioned before this myth is closed is that through most of human existence man only ate once, maybe twice, a day. There is no actual need to eat three times a day and that we do it today is merely a social convention. For thousands of years people have hunted and foraged all day long, expending a lot of energy, and then at the end of the day they'd sit around and eat a very large meal and did just fine.

A lot of people try to muddy the water to sell products and uncover fat loss secrets but you still can't escape the simple truth that fat loss comes down to math and biology: calories in versus calories out combined with controlling insulin, which means eating less.

As I have already noted before, Just so there is no confusion. I'm not saying eating several small meals during the day is bad, the fact is that many people do get benefits from it. Eating small items all day long and having all meals pre-planned does help a lot of people not overeat and stick to their diet. If you are sensitive to low blood sugar then this manner of eating is probably ideal for you.

4: You shouldn't eat just before going to bed because since your body doesn't need the energy while you're sleeping, you will just store everything as fat.

This is a very wide spread myth that is and isn't a myth. I first heard it years ago watching a documentary on sumo wrestlers who would eat a large meal and then take a nap afterwards because they believed "sleep after eating builds bulk".

First, you do need energy while you are sleeping. While you sleep your body is still hard at work keeping you alive and healthy. There are even experts who suggest that you should eat a small meal right before going to bed to keep your blood sugar level while you sleep.

It is true that you will store more of what you eat because when you are asleep there is little to do with all the extra energy you just put in your body. A far greater amount of what you just ate will be stored as fat, however for most people it will even out once you wake up and start the next day.

If you need 2000 calories per day to maintain your current weight and you consume 1000 in the morning and then the other 1000 just before going to sleep you will still have consumed 2000 for that day. Sure, because you didn't consume the full 2000 calories during the day at the exact time your body needed it your body pulled what it needed from energy stored in your cells, but then it put what it didn't need back when you next ate. Again, look at your weight not day by day but rather week to week.

Many people have noticed that if they don't eat before going to sleep they do in fact lose weight. Myself, I've noticed that if I don't eat after 7pm I can easily lose weight but the reason is because I'm in the habit of consuming more calories later at night combined with the fact I'm giving myself a 12-16 hour period of fasting which helps spike my human growth hormone and control my insulin.

5: A calorie is a calorie and that it doesn't matter what you eat as long as you reduce your calories.

The truth of the matter is that not all calories are eＱual and your body does react differently to different things you eat. Simply reducing the number of calories you eat is only a portion of the solution because you also have to control your insulin or you'll be fighting a losing battle.

As we've discussed above, insulin is a hormone your body secretes in response to consuming sugar (carbohydrates) and when insulin enters your blood it allows your body to store the sugars in your cells as energy. The problem with not controlling your insulin levels when you're trying to lose weight is twofold, first insulin represses the effect of the hormone leptin. Leptin is called the "satiety hormone" because it tells your brain that you're full and turns off your hunger. Leptin is produced in your fat cells and when a certain amount enters your bloodstream your brain, specifically your hypothalamus, detects it and creates the feeling of being satisfied. Both insulin and leptin are two of the key hormones that regulate the balance of fat in your body but the problem is that when insulin is high your hypothalamus is unable to accurately gauge the level of leptin in your bloodstream interfering with its effects and preventing you from feeling full and satisfied.

In other words, high insulin levels can prevent you from feeling full and satisfied and keep you feeling hungry despite how much you've eaten. Not only that since your brain is expecting to detect high amounts of leptin but it doesn't is assumes you haven't eaten enough and can strengthen your hunger signals regardless of how much you've eaten.

In addition, since your brain makes you crave foods that contain the nutrients you're lacking if it not detecting enough lepton if often thinks you don't have enough sugar or carbohydrates in your system so it can make you crave fatty and unhealthy foods. This can create a vicious cycle since it is sugar (which carbohydrates get broken down into) that makes insulin levels spike you can eat a bag of candy consuming a lot of sugar and then causing your insulin to spike and then the high amounts of insulin can block the reception of lepton in your brain causing your brain to think you don't have enough sugar in your system, because it can't detect it, and it can make you crave more sugar.

The second problem with not controlling your insulin levels in you want to lose weight is that insulin not only allows you to store energy in your cells but elevated levels of insulin prevent you from pulling energy out of your cells. Let's say you determine that you need to consume 2,000 calories a day to maintain your weight so you figure you'll consume 500 less calories a day so at the end of the week you'll lose one pound of weight. Thinking that a calorie is a calorie you decide it doesn't matter where the calories come from so you decide that you'll get your 1,500 calories that day from chocolate cake.

Since the cake is nothing but sugar and carbohydrates it is going to create a massive spike in your insulin levels so most of that cake is going to get stored as fat. Then the high levels of insulin can prevent your body from detecting the leptin in your blood stream so you can feel very hungry and even crave more sugar. The big problem comes when your body needs that 500 calories you didn't consume that day to maintain your weight. What does it do?

First, it's going to use any glucose found in your bloodstream and then it will use glucose stored in your liver. However, the problem comes when you've done this for a couple days and you're all out of stored glucose in your liver. Normally, since your body needs additional energy it would just pull it out of your fat cells and burn the fat as energy but if you have high insulin levels your body can't access that fat. When your body can't access your fat storage it will have to take energy from where it can access it and that often means protein which means breaking down muscle or other tissue you actually want to keep.

The other thing that happens when your body wants to break down stored fat for energy but can't access it is that it figures that it doesn't have enough stored fat so since it thinks it doesn't have enough energy in will both increase hunger, to get you to consume more energy, and reduce the amount of energy it uses to conserve what it does have.

Your body will end up slowing bodily functions in an effort to conserve energy so you'll find that you're suddenly tired, weak, have a problem concentrating, and pretty much just want to lay down. Since your body is actually doing less your BMR will actually go down which means that you'll be burning less calories!

So it doesn't matter if you eat less calories, if you don't manage your insulin you won't lose fat and can actually end up being more hungry, losing muscle, feeling tired and horrible, and actually slowing your metabolism. However, if you consume foods that cause a very minimal rise in insulin levels now your brain will be able to detect leptin so you'll feel full and your body will be able to access your fat stores so you'll maintain most of your muscle (some lean mass will always be lost when you're losing weight) and the energy to make up your caloric deficit will primarily come from your stored fat which is what you want.

The reason that fasting is great and has been widely practiced for thousands of years is that when you go for a period of about 16-18 hours without eating you burn through all the energy in your bloodstream making your body have to access stored energy. First, it will go to the sugar you have stored in your liver but within 24 to 36 hours without eating that will be depleted and your body will start pulling fat out of your fat stores and your body will go to almost exclusively running itself by burning off your fat.

Since you're not eating anything you have zero insulin response so your body is fully able to access all your fat stores and since you have so much fat being processed in your system your leptin levels skyrocket and you don't feel hungry at all.

Also your human growth hormone rises dramatically during at fast which gives you energy and preserves your lean tissue. The other hormone that increases during fasting is noradrenaline which gives you a big boost of energy. This is why people on fast suddenly, usually around day 4, feel a big surge of energy and during their fast they feel great, are not hungry, and are full of energy. Their body has all the energy they need since they're freely burning their stored body fat and since they're full of leptin, human growth hormone, and noradrenaline they have very high energy levels and think very clearly.

One of the most popular method of fasting is to fast from dinner to dinner so that you get your fasting in but still eat every day. The way this is done is that on Monday you'd stop eating after dinner and not eat again until dinner time on Tuesday. In this way, you'd put in a roughly 24 hour period where you didn't eat so you'd still get the benefits of fasting with that calorie reduction and insulin suppression, but you can eat dinner every day and still be social. Done one or twice a week can have a dramatic effect on your weight loss. To get the biggest result you should stick to foods with a low glycemic index during your eating periods to avoid high insulin levels.

You might be wondering why you haven't heard about the benefits of fasting before and that is because there is no money in it. The food industry is one of the largest and most powerful in the world and the last thing they want you to do is eat less food. Therefore they try to convince you that eating too much isn't the problem you just need to buy special diet food from them and then even eat more food to lose weight by eating 5-6 times a day. Only in America, the land controlled by lobbyists, would the "experts" tell you that you lose weight you have to eat more and more often.

CONCLUSION

First of all, fasting is not starvation. Starvation is the involuntary abstinence from eating forced upon by outside forces; this happens in times of war and famine when food is scarce. Fasting, on the other hand, is voluntary, deliberate, and controlled. Food is readily available but we choose not to eat it due to spiritual, health, or other reasons.

Fasting is as old as mankind, far older than any other forms of diets. Ancient civilizations, like the Greeks, recognized that there was something intrinsically beneficial to periodic fasting. They were often called times of healing, cleansing, purification, or detoxification. Virtually every culture and religion on earth practice some rituals of fasting.

Before the advent of agriculture, humans never ate three meals a day plus snacking in between. We ate only when we found food which could be hours or days apart. Hence, from an evolution standpoint, eating three meals a day is not a requirement for survival. Otherwise, we would not have survived as a species.

Fast forward to the 21st century, we have all forgotten about this ancient practice. After all, fasting is really bad for business! Food manufacturers encourage us to eat multiple meals and snacks a day. Nutritional authorities warn that skipping a single meal will have dire health consequences. Overtime, these messages have been so well-drilled into our heads.

Fasting has no standard duration. It may be done for a few hours to many days to months on end. Intermittent fasting is an eating pattern where we cycle between fasting and regular eating. Shorter fasts of 16-20 hours are generally done more frequently, even daily. Longer fasts, typically 24-36 hours, are done 2-3 times per week. As it happens, we all fast daily for a period of 12 hours or so between dinner and breakfast.

Fasting has been done by millions and millions of people for thousands of years. Is it unhealthy? No. In fact, numerous studies have shown that it has enormous health benefits.

What Happens When We Eat Constantly?

It is best to understand why eating 5-6 meals a day or every few hours (the exact opposite of fasting) may actually do more harm than good. When we eat, we ingest food energy. The key hormone involved is insulin (produced by the pancreas), which rises during meals. Both carbohydrates and protein stimulate insulin. Fat triggers a smaller insulin effect, but fat is rarely eaten alone.

Insulin has two major functions -

First, it allows the body to immediately start using food energy. Carbohydrates are rapidly converted into glucose, raising blood sugar levels. Insulin directs glucose into the body cells to be used as energy. Proteins are broken down into amino acids and excess amino acids may be turned into glucose. Protein does not necessarily raise blood glucose but it can stimulate insulin. Fats have minimal effect on insulin.

Second, insulin stores away excess energy for future use. Insulin converts excess glucose into glycogen and store it in the liver. However, there is a limit to how much glycogen can be stored away. Once the limit is reached, the liver starts turning glucose into fat. The fat is then put away in the liver (in excess, it becomes fatty liver) or fat deposits in the body (often stored as visceral or belly fat).

Therefore, when we eat and snack throughout the day, we are constantly in a fed state and insulin levels remain high. In other words, we may be spending the majority of the day storing away food energy.

What Happens When We Fast?

The process of using and storing food energy that occurs when we eat goes in reverse when we fast. Insulin levels drop, prompting the body to start burning stored energy. Glycogen, the glucose that is stored in the liver, is first accessed and used. After that, the body starts to break down stored body fat for energy.

Thus, the body basically exists in two states - the fed state with high insulin and the fasting state with low insulin. We are either storing food energy or we are burning food energy. If eating and fasting are balanced, then there is no weight gain. If we spend the majority of the day eating and storing energy, there is a good chance that overtime we may end up gaining weight.

Intermittent Fasting Versus Continuous Calorie-Restriction

The portion-control strategy of constant caloric reduction is the most common dietary recommendation for weight loss and type 2 diabetes. For example, the American Diabetes Association recommends a 500-750 kcal/day energy deficit coupled with regular physical activity. Dietitians follow this approach and recommend eating 4-6 small meals throughout the day.

Does the portion-control strategy work in the long-run? Rarely. A cohort study with a 9-year follow-up from the United Kingdom on 176,495 obese individuals indicated that only 3,528 of them succeeded in attaining normal body weight by the end of the study. That is a failure rate of 98%!

Intermittent fasting is not constant caloric restriction. Restricting calories causes a compensatory increase in hunger and worse, a decrease in the body's metabolic rate, a double curse! Because when we are burning fewer calories per day, it becomes increasingly harder to lose weight and much easier to gain weight back after we have lost it. This type of diet puts the body into a "starvation mode" as metabolism revs down to conserve energy. Intermittent fasting does not have any of these drawbacks.

Health Benefits Of Intermittent Fasting may includes;

Increases metabolism leading to weight and body fat loss

Unlike a daily caloric reduction diet, intermittent fasting raises metabolism. This makes sense from a survival standpoint. If we do not eat, the body uses stored energy as fuel so that we can stay alive to find another meal. Hormones allow the body to switch energy sources from food to body fat.

Studies demonstrate this phenomenon clearly. For example, four days of continuous fasting increased Basal Metabolic Rate by 12%. Levels of the neurotransmitter norepinephrine, which prepares the body for action, increased by 117%. Fatty acids in the bloodstream increased over 370% as the body switched from burning food to burning stored fats.

No loss in muscle mass

Unlike a constant calorie-restriction diet, intermittent fasting does not burn muscles as many have feared. In 2010, researchers looked at a group of subjects who underwent 70 days of alternate daily fasting (ate one day and fasted the next). Their muscle mass started off at 52.0 kg and ended at 51.9 kg. In other words, there was no loss of muscles but they did lose 11.4% of fat and saw major improvements in LDL cholesterol and triglyceride levels.

During fasting, the body naturally produces more human growth hormone to preserve lean muscles and bones. Muscle mass is generally preserved until body fat drops below 4%. Therefore, most people are not at risk of muscle-wasting when doing intermittent fasting.

Reverses insulin resistance, type 2 diabetes, and fatty liver

Type 2 diabetes is a condition whereby there is simply too much sugar in the body, to the point that the cells can no longer respond to insulin and take in any more glucose from the blood (insulin resistance), resulting in high blood sugar. Also, the liver becomes loaded with fat as it tries to clear out the excess glucose by converting it to and storing it as fat.

Therefore, to reverse this condition, two things have to happen -

First, stop putting more sugar into the body.
Second, burn the remaining sugar off.

The best diet to achieve this is a low-carbohydrate, moderate-protein, and high-healthy fat diet, also called ketogentic diet. (Remember that carbohydrate raises blood sugar the most, protein to some degree, and fat the least.) That is why a low-carb diet will help reduce the burden of incoming glucose. For some people, this is already enough to reverse insulin resistance and type 2 diabetes. However, in more severe cases, diet alone is not sufficient.

What about exercise? Exercise will help burn off glucose in the skeletal muscles but not all the tissues and organs, including the fatty liver. Clearly, exercise is important, but to eliminate the excess glucose in the organs, there is the need to temporarily "starve" the cells.

Intermittent fasting can accomplish this. That is why historically, people called fasting a cleanse or a detox. It can be a very powerful tool to get rid of all the excesses. It is the fastest way to lower blood glucose and insulin levels, and eventually reversing insulin resistance, type 2 diabetes, and fatty liver.

By the way, taking insulin for type 2 diabetes does not address the root cause of the problem, which is excess sugar in the body. It is true that insulin will drive the glucose away from the blood, resulting in lower blood glucose, but where does the sugar go? The liver is just going to turn it all into fat, fat in the liver and fat in the abdomen. Patients who go on insulin often end up gaining more weight, which worsens their diabetes.

Enhances heart health

Overtime, high blood glucose from type 2 diabetes can damage the blood vessels and nerves that control the heart. The longer one has diabetes, the higher the chances that heart disease will develop. By lowering blood sugar through intermittent fasting, the risk of cardiovascular disease and stroke is also reduced.

In addition, intermittent fasting has been shown to improve blood pressure, total and LDL (bad) cholesterol, blood triglycerides, and inflammatory markers associated with many chronic diseases.

Boosts brain power

Multiple studies demonstrated fasting has many neurologic benefits including attention and focus, reaction time, immediate memory, cognition, and generation of new brain cells. Mice studies also showed that intermittent fasting reduces brain inflammation and prevents the symptoms of Alzheimer's.

What To Expect With Intermittent Fasting

Hunger Goes Down

We normally feel hunger pangs about four hours after a meal. So if we fast for 24 hours, does it mean that our hunger sensations will be six times more severe? Of course not.

Many people are concerned that fasting will result in extreme hunger and overeating. Studies showed that on the day after a one-day fast, there is, indeed, a 20% increase in caloric intake. However, with repeated fasting, hunger and appetite surprisingly decrease.

Hunger comes in waves. If we do nothing, the hunger dissipates after a while. Drinking tea (all kinds) or coffee (with or without caffeine) is often enough to fight it off. However, it is best to drink it black though a teaspoon or two of cream or half-and-half will not trigger much insulin response. Do not use any types of sugar or artificial sweeteners. If necessary, bone broth can also be taken during fasting.

Blood sugar does not crash

Sometimes people worry that blood sugar will fall very low during fasting and they will become shaky and sweaty. This does not actually happen as blood sugar is tightly monitored by the body and there are multiple mechanisms to keep it in the proper range.

During fasting, the body begins to break down glycogen in the liver to release glucose. This happens every night during our sleep.

If we fast for longer than 24-36 hours, glycogen stores become depleted and the liver will manufacture new glucose using glycerol which is a by-product of the breakdown of fat (a process called gluconeogenesis). Apart from using glucose, our brain cells can also use ketones for energy. Ketones are produced when fat is metabolized and they can supply up to 75% of the brain's energy re□uirements (the other 25% from glucose).

The only exception is for those who are taking diabetic medications and insulin. You MUST first consult your doctor as the dosages will probably need to be reduced while you are fasting. Otherwise, if you overmedicate and hypoglycemia develops, which can be dangerous, you must have some sugar to reverse it. This will break the fast and make it counterproductive.

The dawn phenomenon

After a period of fasting, especially in the morning, some people experience high blood glucose. This dawn phenomenon is a result of the circadian rhythm whereby just before awakening, the body secretes higher levels of several hormones to prepare for the upcoming day -

Adrenaline - to give the body some energy
Growth hormone - to help repair and make new protein
Glucagon - to move glucose from storage in the liver to the blood for use as energy
Cortisol, the stress hormone - to activate the body
These hormones peak in the morning hours, then fall to lower levels during the day. In non-diabetics, the magnitude of the blood sugar rise is small and most people will not even notice it. However, for the majority of the diabetics, there can be a noticeable spike in blood glucose as the liver dumps sugar into the blood.

This will happen in extended fasts too. When there is no food, insulin levels stay low while the liver releases some of its stored sugar and fat. This is natural and not a bad thing at all. The magnitude of the spike will decrease as the liver becomes less bloated with sugar and fat.

End Your Weight Loss Frustration by Fasting Away Your Extra Pounds

Weight loss is all about calories in and calorie out. You want to burn more calories than you consume.

By fasting 1 or 2 days per week you dramatically reduce the number of calories consumed and you will lose weight. There are no crazy meal plans to follow but you have to be sensible about your food choices when not fasting. Any weight loss plan has to fit in with your lifestyle and fasting can fit into any lifestyle. It's not restrictive and it doesn't make you resentful. It's actually very liberating and gives you a total sense of control over your body.

Intermittent fasting as a lifestyle will bring about changes that will last a lifetime. As with any weight loss program, start slow and build up. Listen to your body as you start on this journey but don't be tricked into thinking that you are missing out on anything. Many times, especially at first, your body will be going through some withdrawals, and it's important to learn how to differentiate the signals. Look at fasting as an opportunity to break bad eating habits from the past and start a fresh chapter of controlled weight loss and healthy eating. Coupled with an appropriate exercise program fasting can provide you with the weight loss results you have been looking for.

The most important thing to remember about intermittent fasting is that it is not merely a diet plan, but a lifestyle. Look into what intermittent fasting can do for you. Once you start your IF journey, you'll most likely find that you feel fuller longer and can keep the meals you do eat very simple. There are a few different ways you can fast along with a typical meal plan for each day. The combination of nutrients will give you the energy you need to enhance the benefits of your fasting journey. Just make sure to take into account any individual food intolerances, and use this as a guide for your particular health case, and adjust from there.

Does Sleeping At Night Count As Hours Toward The Fast?

Yes, it does. So, for example, if you have a protein shake right before bed, then wake up eight hours later, you're already eight hours into your fast with only eight more to reach your goal of 16.

What Should I Eat Or Drink While Intermittent Fasting?

Obviously, you don't eat anything or consume any calories during your fasting hours—simply put, don't eat any food or shakes. Water, of course, is perfectly fine. Other than that, opt for zero-calorie, unsweetened beverages. My personal favorites include black coffee—with no milk, cream, sugar, butter (for you Bulletproof-coffee fans), or anything else in it—and plain, unsweetened teas like black tea or green tea.

When it comes to calorie-free drinks with artificial sweeteners (like flavored waters and diet soda), there's a bit of uncertainty. There's some evidence to show that some artificial sweeteners cause an insulin response, which would then blunt your ability to burn fat and contradict the point of being in a fasted state.

To be on the safe side, I recommend not drinking artificially sweetened beverages during a fast. If you're absolutely dying for something other than water or plain coffee or tea during the last few hours of a fast, opt for a sparkling water that's very lightly flavored with something like natural lime.

Do I Need To Cram A Day's Worth Of Meals Into Eight Hours?

Regarding the "feeding window," (AKA the joyous time during which you get to eat) you want to reach the same calorie and macronutrient totals as you were before—provided you were already on a solid diet plan that corresponded to your goals, of course.

You definitely don't want to undereat during your feeding window, or you'll compromise your performance in the gym and your ability to build or maintain muscle mass. Get in all of your nutrients, particularly protein.

In theory, you'll be eating the same number of calories and macros per day, just with a different meal schedule than a typical eat-every-few-hours nutrition plan. Of course, you can always tweak calories and macros if and when your physi☐ue and weight loss goals change.

Final tips and tricks about Fasting

Don't freak out! Stop wondering: "can I fast 15 hours instead of 16?" or "what if I eat an apple during my fasted period, will that ruin everything?" Relax. Your body is a complex piece of machinery and learns to adapt. Everything is not as cut and dry as you think.

If you want to eat breakfast one day but not another, that's okay. If you are going for optimal aesthetic or athletic performance, I can see the need to be more rigid in your discipline, but otherwise…freaking chill out and don't stress over minutiae! Don't let perfect be the enemy of good.

Consider fasted walks in the morning. I found these to be very helpful in reducing body fat, and also gave my day a great start to clear my mind and prepare for the day. Simply wake up and go for a mile walk. Maybe you could even start walking to Mordor?

Listen to your body during workouts. If you get light headed, make sure you are consuming enough water. If you notice a significant drop in performance, make sure you are eating enough calories (especially fats and protein) during your feasting window. And if you feel severely "off," pause your workout. Give yourself permission to EASE into intermittent fasting and fasted workouts. This is especially true if you are an endurance athlete.

Expect funny looks if you spend a lot of mornings with breakfast eaters. A few weeks back I had a number of friends staying with me, and they were all completely dumbfounded when I told them I didn't eat breakfast anymore. I tried to explain it to them but received a bunch of blank stares. Breakfast has become so engrained (zing!) in our culture that NOT eating it sounds crazy. You will get weird looks from those around you…embrace it. I still go to brunch or sit with friends, I just drink black coffee and enjoy conversation.

Stay busy. If you are just sitting around thinking about how hungry you are, you'll be more likely to struggle with this. For that reason, I time my fasting periods for maximum efficiency and minimal discomfort:

My first few hours of fasting come after consuming a MONSTER meal, where the last thing I want to think about is eating.

When I'm sleeping: 8 of my 16 hours are occupied by sleeping. Tough to feel hungry when I'm dreaming about becoming a Jedi. When I'm busy: After waking up, 12 hours of my fasting is already done. I spend three hours doing my best work (while drinking a cup of black coffee), and then comes my final hour of fasting: training.

Zero-calorie beverages are okay. I drink green tea in the morning for my caffeine kick while writing. If you want to drink water, black coffee, or tea during your fasted period, that's okay. Remember, don't overthink it – keep things simple! Dr. Rhonda Patrick over at FoundMyFitness believes that a fast should stop at the first consumption of anything other than water, so experiment yourself and see how your body responds.

If you want to put milk in your coffee, or drink diet soda occasionally while fasting, I'm not going to stop you. Remember, we're going for consistency and habit-building here – if milk or cream in your coffee makes life worth living, don't deprive yourself.

There are MUCH bigger fish to fry with regards to getting healthy than a few calories here and there during a fast. 80% adherence that you stick with for a year is better than 100% adherence that you abandon after a month because it was too restrictive. If you're trying to get to a minimum bodyfat percentage, you'll need to be more strict – until then, however, do what allows you to stay compliant!

Track your results, listen to your body

Concerned about losing muscle mass? Keep track of your strength training routines and see if you are getting stronger.

Buy a cheap set of body fat calipers and keep track of your body fat composition.

Track your calories, and see how your body changes when eating the same amount of food, but condensed into a certain window.

Give Intermittent Fasting a try

If you're ready to give intermittent fasting a try, consider skipping breakfast, make sure you stop eating and drinking anything but water three hours before you go to sleep, and restrict your eating to an 8-hour (or less) time frame every day. In the 6-8 hours that you do eat, have healthy protein, minimize your carbs like pasta, bread, and potatoes and exchange them for healthful fats like butter, eggs, avocado, coconut oil, olive oil and nuts — essentially the very fats the media and "experts" tell you to avoid.

This will help shift you from carb burning to fat burning mode. Once your body has made this shift, it is nothing short of magical as your cravings for sweets, and food in general, rapidly normalizes and your desire for sweets and junk food radically decreases if not disappears entirely.

Remember it takes a few weeks, and you have to do it gradually, but once you succeed and switch to fat burning mode, you'll be easily able to fast for 18 hours and not feel hungry. The "hunger" most people feel is actually cravings for sugar, and these will disappear as if by magic, once you successfully shift over to burning fat instead.

Another phenomenal side effect/benefit that occurs is that you will radically improve the beneficial bacteria in your gut. Supporting healthy gut bacteria, which actually outnumber your cells 10 to one, is one of the most important things you can do to improve your immune system so you won't get sick, or get coughs, colds and flus. You will sleep better, have more energy, have increased mental clarity and concentrate better. Essentially every aspect of your health will improve as your gut flora becomes balanced.

Inaddition, based on my own phenomenal experience with intermittent fasting, I believe it's one of the most powerful ways to shift your body into fat burning mode and improve a wide variety of biomarkers for disease. The effects can be further magnified by exercising while in a fasted state. Clearly, it's another powerful tool in your box to help you and your family take control of your health, and an excellent way to take your fitness to the next level.